G000167773

THE EFFECTS OF
Yoga on
Hypertension

The Effects of
Yoga on
Hypertension

Dr Swami Shankardevananda
MBBS (Sydney)

Under the Guidance of
Swami Satyananda Saraswati

Bihar School of Yoga, Munger, Bihar, India

First published 1978
Second edition 1984
Reprinted 1998

© 1978, 1998

Copyright reserved by Bihar School of Yoga.

Publisher: Swami Satyasangananda Saraswati,
Honorary Secretary, Bihar School of Yoga,
Ganga Darshan, Munger, Bihar, India.

ISBN: 81-85787-27-1

Printer: Bhargava Bhushan Press, Trilochan,
Varanasi, UP, India.

SWAMI SIVANANDA SARASWATI

Swami Sivananda was born at Patta-
madai, Tamil Nadu, in 1887. After
serving as a medical doctor in Malaya,
he renounced his practice, went to
Rishikesh and was initiated into
Dashnami Sannyasa in 1924 by Swami
Vishwananda Saraswati. He toured
extensively throughout India, inspir-
ing people to practise yoga and lead
a divine life. He founded the Divine
Life Society at Rishikesh in 1936, the
Sivananda Ayurvedic Pharmacy in
1945, the Yoga Vedanta Forest
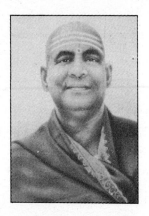
Academy in 1948 and the Sivananda Eye Hospital in 1957.
During his lifetime he guided thousands of disciples and
aspirants all over the world and authored over 200 books.

SWAMI SATYANANDA SARASWATI

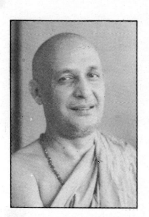
Swami Satyananda was born at
Almora, Uttar Pradesh, in 1923. In
1943 he met Swami Sivananda in
Rishikesh and adopted the Dashnami
Sannyasa way of life. In 1955 he left
his guru's ashram to live as a wandering mendicant and later founded the
International Yoga Fellowship in 1963
and the Bihar School of Yoga in 1964.
Over the next 20 years he toured inter-
nationally and authored over 80
books. In 1987 he founded Sivananda
Math, a charitable institution for rural
development, and the Yoga Research Foundation. In 1988
he renounced his mission, adopting kshetra sannyasa, and
now lives as a paramahamsa sannyasin.

SWAMI NIRANJANANANDA SARASWATI

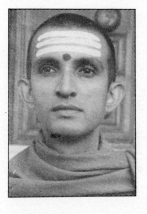

Swami Niranjanananda was born at Rajnandgaon, Madhya Pradesh in 1960. At the age of 4 he joined the Bihar School of Yoga and was initiated into Dashnami Sannyasa at the age of 10. From 1971 he travelled overseas and toured many countries for the next 11 years. In 1983 he was recalled to India and appointed President of Bihar School of Yoga. During the following 11 years he guided the development of Ganga Darshan, Sivananda Math and the Yoga Research Foundation. In 1990 he was initiated as a Paramahamsa and in 1993 anointed Preceptor in succession to Swami Satyananda. Bihar Yoga Bharati was founded under his direction in 1994. He has authored over 20 books and guides national and international yoga programs.

Foreword

by Dr Shreenivas MD*
11th June, 1978

The primary or essential hypertension, *hyperpiesia*, is earned and acquired rather than inherited or bestowed. Although the tendency to it may be a gift of the genes, the disorder is largely psychosomatic.

The management of the hypertensive patient is bedevilled by problems. The clinical definition of abnormal limits of blood pressure are illusory and vague. There are surprisingly individual and racial differences of tolerance which are not yet fully determined.

One of my patients, an Anglo-Indian lady in her 50's was able to look after herself with a blood pressure of about 320 mm of Hg systolic and 260 mm of Hg diastolic. Still she ultimately died, years later, of congestive heart failure and auricular fibrillation.

During a statistical study of the 'Normal Blood Pressure Range in Nepal and Bihar', I found that the highest (around 140–150/80–90 mm Hg) blood pressure range was exhibited by non-vegetarian, well-fed, urban, well-built, responsible males in the age-group of 21–30 years. Many extremely

*Director-Professor Indira Gandhi Institute of Cardiovascular Diseases, Bihar, Patna (retd); Director Yoga Research Institute, Patna; Ella-Lyman Cabot Fellow (Harvard, USA); Haskell Fellow (Kansas, USA); Professor and Head of Department of Medicine, Patna Medical College Hospital (retd); Member of the IYFM Research Coordinating Centre, Bihar School of Yoga, Munger, Bihar, India.

vii

high readings were recorded among post-graduate students of universities in Bihar and among soldiers of the Nepalese regiment. This range of blood pressure was exceeded only by villagers over 80 years of age. In Nepal the highest blood pressure (166/101 mm Hg) was encountered among the businessmen and the Government servants (excluding the well-to-do and easy going Ranas). The lowest blood pressure was recorded in the Tamangs, Lamas and Bhotias (104\56 mm Hg average). People with systolic blood pressure above 140 mm Hg and diastolic blood pressure above 90 mm Hg constituted only 20% of the total healthy population in Bihar and about 30% of the total healthy population of Nepal. It was felt that worry was one of the major factors behind hypertension. Age, sex, body build, diet, tobacco and climate are relatively less important. It was also apparent that the problem of blood pressure in society must be tackled quite early and that one should start working with teenagers. In order to derive maximum benefits from yoga, it too should be inculcated by the young.

There is no 'ideal' anti-hypertensive drug available. They are accompanied by many kinds of drawbacks and contra-indications, some of them quite serious and severe. Their short and long term effects are unpredictable and their 'toxicity' may create iatrogenic illnesses rather than alleviate suffering. Worst of all may be their baneful influences on the mind and the autonomic nervous system and the enzymatic and chemical mediators. The ganglion-blockers, the sympatholytics, the enzyme inhibitors, the depressants, seem to ransack normal physiology, gripping it and clutching on it, so that it becomes cluttered, wrecked and ruined. The victim loses control of his own body mechanisms and is no longer master of himself. It is unfortunate to thus become unarmed and uncloaked, to be deprived of one's freedom, and to be forced into a situation of such surreptitious servitude, of unmitigated dependence on drugs.

Apart from the use of drugs there are other well-known measures which significantly lower the blood pressure. For example the loss of weight, low salt intake, a vegetarian diet consisting of rice and fruits, the use of garlic; and the riddance from lapping anxieties and lacerating agitations. The practice of yoga may verily be one such additional measure. It is easy to learn, universally acceptable, economical and harmless. It leaves a person in full control of mind and body while mopping up even hidden traces of stress and strain.

It has been proved by the Yoga Research Institute at Patna that the lowering of blood pressure is easier and more spectacular with yoga than with simple rest and tranquilizers (e.g. Diazepam).

Yoga improves physical, mental, psychic and spiritual health. It makes the physiological reflexes, reactions and responses more alert, sensitive and subtle. It exercises and energizes the various systems of the body. The asanas are so designed that their effects may reach to the very ends of the peripheral nerve tips, even to the tiniest and finest and most slender capillaries, to the *vasa nervorum* and the *vasa vasorum* and the nutrient arteries which pierce and ply through the hard bones to supply the marrow, and even to each of the individual cells wherever they may be located in the body.

Yoga helps to change the lifestyle of the practitioner. We learn to adjust and adapt to changing life situations and circumstances and to accept the environment stoically but wisely and in good humour. It awakens man to the realities of existence, infuses hope and courage, and rekindles zest and zeal. There is no passive acceptance of fate or destiny; the yogi does not sit moping, repenting, complaining, carping and condemning. He is glad to take up the gauntlet and to accept the challenge. He is part of the Cosmic Conjuror and is not cowering under stress or cringing before strain.

Yoga is a definite and precise breakthrough in the prevention and treatment of hypertension. It may be used alone or in conjunction with other measures including drugs. While drugs may remove the prick, yoga removes the thorn. The great merit of this book is that its approach is rational and objective. It deftly portrays the problems involved and cites precise reasons for the inclusion of yoga as an additional and alternative therapeutic measure. The medical and clinical aspects are well covered. The facts are simply and succinctly stated. The steps to be followed are clear.

The erudite author has covered the subject exceptionally well. He has rendered yeoman's service to mankind by publishing such a useful and magnificent treatise on health and hygiene pertaining to one of the most common diseases afflicting mankind.

Yoga is to be cultured. It has to be incorporated in our daily lives and accepted as an essential ingredient and as an integral part of our routine and life pattern. The technique should be avidly pursued and implemented. The human being must be saved from the ravages of hypertension, secured from the dangers of drugs, and protected from the annoyance and drudgery of perpetual reconciliations, compromises and restrictions imposed by specialists.

Yoga, the alternative anti-hypertensive regimen so aptly and avowedly advocated by the author, is at once authentic and ingenious.

Contents

Preface

Hypertension is one of many psychosomatic diseases which can be treated through a combination of yoga and traditional medicine. This disease is a symbol of other maladies from which mankind currently suffers and which cause seemingly endless suffering. The root cause of all disease is the same: ignorance of our true nature and lack of awareness of who we really are.

This book will help you gain a better understanding of your physical, pranic, mental, psychic and spiritual bodies. Once you understand these you will begin to kindle the flames of peace and good health. You will gain the strength to prevent disease from forming.

This manual grew from the smaller *Yogic Management of High Blood Pressure*, as a result of the demand for an alternative to the methods available for *cure* of high blood pressure. It is intended to bridge the various healing systems and to show people that there is a cure for high blood pressure (hypertension), and a way to break the vicious cycle of disease, no matter what it has been given.

Thanks must go to Dr Swami Vivekananda MBBS, MANZCP, DPM, for critical editing, and Dr Shreenivas MD, Director of the Yoga Research Institute, Patna, India, whose guidance and experimental work were most helpful.

Preface to the Second Edition

Hypertension is one of the most common diseases and, through the agency of the press and media, more and more people are becoming aware of this. The threat of heart disease and blood pressure is so great that, in some countries, the very mention of these dreaded illnesses is enough to cause palpitations and a rise in blood pressure.

Since this book was first published, there has been a significant increase in the number of people turning to yoga, meditation, relaxation, biofeedback and other techniques designed to reduce the effects of stress upon the body. Indeed, with the growing awareness of the need for more exercise, a good diet and relaxation, especially amongst the sedentary occupations and business populations, recent medical journals have announced a significant decrease in deaths from heart attack. This is very encouraging.

However, at the same time as we are prolonging the quantity of our life span, we must also think about its quality. For this, yoga is one of the best means to ensure a full, active and happy life.

This book is aimed at several groups of people who are concerned and involved with hypertension.

Doctors should regard this text as a simple outline of the medical/physiological view of hypertension with the yogic view interspersed. This aims to broaden and deepen the purely physical approach that most doctors are taught and accustomed to use and expands their perception of the disease into the more subtle energies and mental side as well. Doctors can then recommend yoga to their patients, either referring them to an ashram or a competent yoga teacher. Even better, the doctors can learn yoga themselves and then teach it to others.

Yoga teachers who wish to use yoga in a semi-therapeutic situation, must be aware of the total picture of the disease, the dangers they may meet and the correct application and modulation of yogic asana, pranayama and relaxation practices to suit the individual needs of their students. In this regard they would be wise to stick to a simple sadhana and work with a competent yogic guru as well as with a broad-minded doctor who will help them to understand what disease they are dealing with, its extent and severity, and any possible dangers.

The patient with hypertension should use this book to guide him into both theoretical knowledge and practical application under expert guidance. A deeper understanding of hypertension is important if we are to change, grow and heal ourselves because we must first become aware of those factors in our attitude to life and to ourselves (most importantly), as well as in our lifestyle, which are causing our blood pressure to rise. Attitude is ultimately most important because it powers and directs our mental energies in either a positive or negative direction.

Knowledge of the layout of the circulatory system, its links with the rest of the body and mind, and how it goes wrong, will definitely speed up the healing process once it has been initiated through yoga and relaxation. This book will then serve as a guide throughout the course of the healing process which can take anywhere from a few months to years.

People who do not have hypertension but who wish to know more about the disease, either because of interest, or because they may be in a situation in which hypertension is likely, for example a high pressure business or job, should thoroughly go through the book. Not only will they gain in general knowledge, but if they apply the suggestions to their lives, will prevent the scourge of hypertension. This is important because hypertension is so insidious that often it is upon us before we know it.

Because hypertension is relatively symptom-free in the beginning (especially pain-free) we tend to ignore it until the complications set in or until the prospect of a reduced lifetime filled with pain, disease and endless medical bills, wakes us up to the fact that we have to do something about our situation. We all know that prevention is better than cure and that early cases are easier to deal with than older, more complicated situations. However, few of us know how to prevent disease or what to do when it occurs because we are sadly uninformed or misinformed. For example, there are many misconceptions about yoga. However, even when we do know, the tragedy of man is that he does not act.

This book has been modified, especially in the practice sections, in order to clarify and underline certain important aspects of the yogic approach to hypertension. The importance of breathing, breath awareness and the need for consistent, determined, repetitive practice, has been highlighted in order to enhance the power of yoga.

Often, when we fail to get the results we desire, whether it be in yoga or anything, we tend to blame the system itself rather than recognizing whether we have been making some mistake or not, or whether more effort is necessary.

It is our fervent prayer that all those who read this book and start on the path of yoga will eradicate the scourge of hypertension for themselves and pass on the message to those unfortunate enough not to know about yoga and what it can do to uplift and transform our lives.

Dr Swami Shankardevananda
Munger, 1983

Introduction

Our body-mind complex is a marvel of creation both intricate and subtle in design. Man, who inhabits it, is finding out new and astounding facts about his inner workings, facts which are helping to open up his awareness, understanding and knowledge of himself. This knowledge is leading him out of the mire of disease and suffering to a state of better health and longevity.

Why is this apparent marvel of creation so prone to illnesses such as high blood pressure? What is the ultimate cause of disease? These are questions which modern science, despite its great technological advances, is still unable to answer. Yoga, however, can give an insight into these problems helping us to reach our own conclusion through meditative experience of the higher reaches of awareness.

The science of yoga offers a theoretical construct for the workings of body and mind and their malfunction in disease, as well as the practices to correct imbalance and help us gain better health and realization. Yoga provides a path to the cure of high blood pressure but it is you, the seeker of health, who must tread it. With increased knowledge of the body, its energy systems, the mind, the soul, and their inter-relationships, we can learn to live more harmonious, better integrated lives, and health is a natural consequence of this.

To be healthy, mentally and physically, one must know the body-mind complex, its needs and requirements, just as a car requires a good driver as well as servicing, oiling, petrol, grease, tyre adjustment and so on. People are sick because they do not know their bodies and minds, what they need and how to keep them properly. Yoga is designed to help us maintain this body-mind vehicle in top running condition for as long as possible so that life can be joyful, free and fulfilling.

Yoga offers a sublime philosophy and a practical means to realize it, and doctors are now finding within the broad scope of yogic philosophy many solutions to existing dilemmas facing both doctor and patient. Modern medicine has discovered the jewel of yoga and is combining methods of yoga with medical treatment. The courtship of medicine and yoga is complete; now each will have to realize the other's greatness.

Yoga is union, and in terms of healing, yoga implies the coming together of all systems and pathies; allopathy, homeopathy, chiropractic, ayurveda, polypathy, and so on. The doctor or healer should have all these systems at his disposal, selecting the relevant points from each, and distilling from this mixture the pure essence, the renowned philosopher's stone. Yoga is, therefore, a matrix, or framework on which to unravel the old and weave the new, building up a more ideal system to cope with the problems of our modern world, of which hypertension is only one.

Through the combination of medicine and yoga, both doctor and patient can come to a better understanding of the disease process involved in hypertension and so learn from experience, growing and maturing within. In this way we become not only physically healthy, but gain a dynamic personality, mental and emotional stability, and deeper wisdom and insight. This is real healing which fulfils the function of the doctor (from the Latin *docere*, 'to teach') and lifts the patient into the higher spheres, towards union with higher consciousness.

Cause

Circulatory System

It is hoped that through this simple account of the action of the heart and circulatory system you can build up a picture in your imagination of what is actually going on in your body. From this understanding you will be able to sensitize your awareness of the body processes.

A serious desire to overcome hypertension, or to lift your awareness to greater heights, begins with such an understanding of the body. It helps to develop awareness of the functions within the physical and mental frames. A vivid visualization of these internal functions is essential in gaining good health and to the success of the higher practices of yoga. This allows you to subsequently maintain your health and to prevent future disease through the process of strengthening the mind.

Yoga is a scientific system of self-discovery, self-maintenance and self-cure. To know the internal workings of the body from the medical and the yogic points of view is an advantage, but to experience the practical results of this knowledge is the outcome of regular practice of yoga techniques. The wonders contained within your own frame are endless. Yoga is the means to their discovery.

General concepts
The physiology of the circulatory system is very complex. This system feeds every cell of the body with life-giving fluid

containing oxygen and nutrients. It is not important that you understand all the complexities of this system. It is important that you have in your mind's eye a picture, whether symbolic or actual, of those mechanisms that deliver blood throughout the body and which, when imbalanced, cause hypertension. In this way you will be better equipped to manipulate your own body and effect a cure.

The circulatory system is composed of the heart, blood vessels and the blood itself. The heart is like the trunk of the tree. From this central point branches radiate out into the body, each getting smaller and smaller until finally they become minute and merge into the cell structure of the organ they are feeding. They then grow larger again,

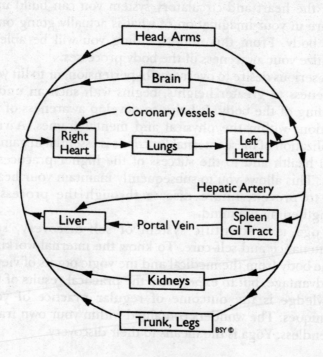

The Circulatory System

4

following the same general route they took to the organ, but this time they are heading back towards the heart. In this way we have two trees from the same root, shadowing each other. They are the same size but vary a little in structure. The main difference is the direction of blood flow within.

In this way a system of feeding the body cells, the basic units of the body organs, and of removing waste and impurities has been established. This is a vital system to the life of the body. If any part should not receive blood for any reason it will die. Thus the circulatory system must be maintained in the best possible health.

If a part breaks down it interferes with the function of all body systems, upsetting the order, balance and harmony of regulation, and leads on to serious disease. This happens in high blood pressure, where a narrowing of the arterioles (part of the system leading from the heart) prevents adequate nutrition of organs.

Blood

Blood is a highly complex liquid. It is alive with cells floating in what is basically water. Blood comprises about eight percent of the body weight in the adult and this usually means a volume of about five to six litres. Blood is composed of:

- *Plasma*: This is the fluid that carries the cells. It is ninety percent water and contains organic solids (such as proteins), hormones, antibodies and enzymes, as well as waste material, foodstuff, salts and respiratory gases.
- *Cells*: There are two groups of cells, the red blood cells and the white blood cells. The red cells carry oxygen. The white cells are important in the body's defences against pus-forming organisms, allergies, and acute and chronic infections. They attack foreign material that gets past the first defence system of the body. There are also cells called platelets which help the blood clot.

Blood flows through tubes (blood vessels) under pressure; that is, blood pressure. This pressure arises because of the four following mechanisms:

5

1. *Cardiac output*: The heart pumps blood into the larger vessels which are like elastic and exert some resistance to the flow. The amount of blood pumped into these vessels determines, to a degree, the pressure within the vessels.
2. *Peripheral resistance*: The degree of resistance met by the pumped blood when it approaches smaller vessels towards the extremities of the body. If these vessels are constricted there is a greater amount of resistance than if they are open. This is the fundamental cause of hypertension.
3. *Viscosity of blood*: Thicker blood is harder to pump. This means that the greater the viscosity or thickness, the more the blood pressure rises.
4. *Volume of blood*: A larger volume inside the closed system of vessels also increases blood pressure.

The blood being pushed into the smaller arteries is under a constant state of tension because the heart is pumping into this closed system. Increase of the pressure increases the tension of the vessel walls, and an excess of this pressure causes hypertension.

The blood continuously flows, moving at a rapid pace inside the vessels. If you concentrate on this movement you can gradually build up your awareness of the flow of blood. It is well worth your while to sit down for a few minutes and try to become aware of all the different movements taking place just under your skin. The system of vessels and blood nourishes the tissues, bringing oxygen. Close your eyes. Relax. Let your awareness float along your bloodstream.

Blood vessels

These are the tubes which convey blood away from the heart and bring it back again. They organize the flow of blood so that every organ, no matter how far away from the heart, receives its share. Otherwise the organs closest to the heart would receive the best and purest blood, contaminate it and then send it to organs further away. In this way the body would not function efficiently. The blood vessels are called arteries, veins and capillaries.

6

1. *Arteries:* These are elastic or muscular-walled, tubular structures of three types.
   a) *Elastic arteries* are the large conducting vessels near the heart. They can expand when the heart contracts because of the elastic tissue in their walls. In this way they store energy, for while the heart refills after contraction, the arteries recoil and propel the blood along. The blood flows in a steady stream and not by stops and starts, ensuring smooth blood flow. The best example of an elastic artery is the *aorta*, the biggest artery of the body which leads directly from the heart.
   b) *Muscular arteries* are distributing arteries which lead to organs. At a certain stage the elastic arteries, which have been getting gradually smaller, lose their elastic property and become muscular. The more muscular tissue content an artery has in its walls, the more its carrying capacity is under the direct control of the nervous system.
   c) *Arterioles* are smaller muscular vessels which regulate the flow of blood into the capillary beds within the organ itself. These vessels have the capacity to shut down the flow, if necessary, so as to redirect blood into areas where there is a greater need. It is here that blood meets the greatest peripheral resistance.

   Arteries have a pulse that you can feel. The best known of these pulses is at the wrist on the thumb side, the radial pulse, inside the radial artery. The pulse occurs every time the heart contracts. In the normal adult it occurs sixty to ninety times every minute. With age or with early hardening of the arteries the walls may lose their capacity to stretch and recoil under pressure, increasing the pressure inside the vessels.
2. *Capillaries*: These are the smallest of the blood vessels. They have very thin walls, which are only one cell thick so that oxygen and blood can diffuse into the surrounding cells, and wastes can be eliminated.
3. *Veins*: The capillaries unite to form venules (small veins) which convey blood back into the larger veins and then

7

to the heart. These larger veins have valves along their length which prevent blood flowing backward, although the largest veins which feed directly into the heart have no valves. The great veins are called the *superior vena cava* and *inferior vena cava,* or *S.V.C.* and *I.V.C.*

Blood flow

The body has a lot of work to do in getting the blood to travel the long distance from the bottom of the feet to the heart, approximately five feet from the ground. To do this several mechanisms are employed:

- The force of *gravity*, which helps blood to flow from the head downwards.
- The *respiratory pump*, which sucks blood up into the chest. This action results from suction created by the difference in pressure between the abdominal cavity and chest cavity.
- The *muscle pump* or the contraction of the muscles of the legs and body which serve to push the blood up in the direction of the heart.
- The *cardiac pump* caused by the pressure of the blood being pushed out of the heart contributes to the return because the system is closed.
- *Back pressure* on the valves in the veins causes them to shut so that blood only flows towards the heart.
- *Volume* of blood and *tone* of the blood vessels is important. The tone is the degree of constriction or dilation of the smaller vessels. If the vessels are too dilated then the blood pools at the bottom of the body away from the brain, and fainting can occur. When a person faints he falls, allowing the blood to run into the brain, reoxygenating it for a quick recovery.

The rate of flow is fastest in the large blood vessels and slowest in small blood vessels. This is because the large blood vessels branch into an enormous number of smaller ones and thus distribute the blood over a huge area. It is like a fast flowing river feeding into the sea. The sea is the capillary network. This serves the best interests of the body because the slow flow of blood in the capillaries facilitates the exchange of nutrients for wastes.

Systems of vessels

There are two main systems of blood vessels in the body. One is the *systemic circulation* which feeds the body as a whole. The other is the *pulmonary circulation* which feeds into the lungs. The systemic circulation takes oxygenated blood from the lungs and distributes it to the body. The pulmonary system takes the deoxygenated blood to the lungs for reoxygenation.

The heart

In yogic literature the heart is not only the centre of the circulatory system but also the centre for compassion. It is the physical manifestation of the psychic centre called *anahata chakra*, the subtle heart of our being.

In contrast to yoga, which teaches a science of mind, modern medicine is still looking for the mind, and believes it to reside in the brain. However, the ancient yogis and rishis located the mind, or the higher mind, in the heart. This is the abode of the *jivatma*, of consciousness itself. Within the physical heart is the *sinus node*, the point from which the spark of energy is released that initiates the contractions of the heart and coordinates its activity. This point corresponds to that point said in the ancient scriptures to be the dwelling place of jivatma, a few inches to the right of the centre of the body. There is, as yet, no scientific theory to account for the miracle of the sinus node, how it functions without rest for the whole of our life. It is an enigma that waits to be solved.

At the physical level the heart is mainly composed of muscle. This muscle is lined on both sides by membrane which is lubricated so that the heart moves easily. The muscle of the heart is really two pumps in one. It is divided in half by a middle wall; each half is completely separated from the other. The right side receives deoxygenated blood from the

9

body and sends it to the lungs. The left side receives oxygenated blood and sends it to the body. Both halves are again divided in half within themselves. The upper chamber on each side is called the right and left *atrium* respectively. Below these are the right and left *ventricles*.

The heart operates through these four different chambers and creates a biphasic cycle. There is an active

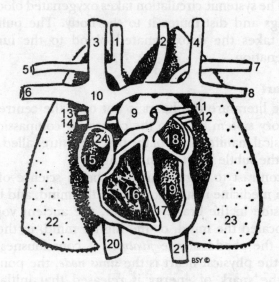

The Heart and the Seat of the Soul

1. Right carotid artery (to head)
2. Left carotid artery (to head)
3. Right jugular vein (from head)
4. Left jugular vein (from head)
5. Right subclavian artery (to arm)
6. Right subclavian vein (from arm)
7. Left subclavian artery (to arm)
8. Left subclavian vein (from arm)
9. Aorta
10. Superior vena cava
11. Left pulmonary artery (to lungs)
12. Left pulmonary vein (from lungs)
13. Right pulmonary artery (to lungs)
14. Right pulmonary vein (from lungs)
15. Right atrium
16. Right ventricle
17. Interventricular septum
18. Left atrium
19. Left ventricle
20. Inferior vena cava
21. Aorta
22. Right lung
23. Left lung
24. Sinus node and Seat of the Soul

10

contracting phase called *systole*, and a passive filling phase called *diastole*. These two halves comprise one beat of the heart. There are between sixty and ninety beats per minute.

An isolated heart cell beats at a rate of about forty cycles per minute. When two cells are placed together they both beat at approximately the same rate but not in phase, as long as they do not touch one another. It has been found experimentally that when the two cells touch they start to function as one cell and beat synchronously. This is what happens in the heart. The sinus node, or pacemaker, however, which initiates contraction of the heart, beats at a faster rate and sends out a current of energy that makes all the other heart cells contract together. In this way, the sinus node makes the heart act as a whole, and thus it functions properly. The brain and its connections to the heart only regulate the speed and coordinate it with the rest of the body according to need.

The heart is a most amazing organ. When it functions properly it is both a gracefully beautiful and an efficient pump, powerful and rhythmic in action. When pressure is needed it will increase the force of its contraction and its speed; similarly it slows its pace when necessary. It seems to have a life of its own, sitting in the middle of the body, beating constantly, evenly, without interruption, every day of the week, every week of the year and every year of our lives. It is a powerful worker and a true karma yogi, never tiring or giving up.

The heart cycle

The heart pumps in a cyclic fashion. This cycle is divided into two phases. One is an active phase called systole, and gives rise to the phase of the blood pressure called the systolic blood pressure. During this phase the heart contracts and increases blood pressure. The other phase is passive or filling, and is called diastole. In this phase the pressure within the blood vessels is at its lowest and represents the pressure that exists as a baseline. This base is the tension

11

that exists within the vessels when the heart is not contracting. It is the more important of the two levels to the doctor when he is measuring your blood pressure because it best represents the state of the autonomic nervous system. This system is responsible for maintaining the tone of your vessels.

The heart pumps blood. When it is actually pumping it is said to be in systole. After each pumping action, or contraction, the heart is emptied and the blood moves into the arteries, which pushes the rest of the blood in the vessels along. The resting stage starts. During this stage the work of propelling the blood is now done by the elastic recoil of the large arteries. Blood is prevented from flowing back into the heart by special valves which permit flow in only one direction. During the resting diastolic period the upper chambers again fill with blood. When they are full they contract, sending the blood into the lower chambers, the ventricles. When the ventricles fill, the muscle contracts, pushing blood out. This stretches the walls of the elastic arteries.

Nervous control of the heart

In the heart, contraction occurs because of a tiny piece of modified muscle tissue called the sinus node. This node is a small round piece of nervous tissue inside the right atrium. It sends out an impulse that makes muscle tissue contract. This impulse travels down the atria to the point of contact with the ventricles. At this stage the atria have contracted.

At the junction between the atria and ventricles there is another modified piece of muscle tissue that slows the impulse down. This is called the A-V node (atrioventricular node). The delay gives the ventricles just enough time to fill to the optimum volume. Then the impulse travels down a special system of conduits, designed to carry current speedily to all the cells of the heart in an ordered and systematic fashion. The cells at the top contract just a little before those at the bottom. In this way blood is pushed along and expelled. The whole cycle takes about 0.8 of a second when the heart rate is seventy-five beats per minute.

The rate of contraction is controlled by the autonomic nervous system which is in two parts. The sympathetic component speeds up the heart while the parasympathetic component slows it down. The sympathetic system prepares the body to face the external environment and any stressful situations, whereas the parasympathetic system allows the body to relax. We usually swing between these two components depending on need. If you are tense your heart beats faster, blood vessels contract and the work load of the heart is increased. This leads to higher blood pressure. The breath is also increased to meet the demand for more oxygen, and most people will find that on closer examination of the whole body they are generally tense and the abdominal muscles have tightened. There is a distinct relationship between the heart and the lungs, and this in turn is related to the mental state, which is mediated by the autonomic nervous system.

When the mind is tense it switches on the sympathetic component. This causes the heart and lungs to function as a team, one bringing more oxygen into the body so that the other can carry it to the cells via the blood stream. Emotional and psychic factors play a very important part in regulation of the heart. Fear and excitement speed it up through their effect on the brain which sends impulses to the autonomic nervous system controller, the *hypothalamus*. Other factors, such as a need for oxygen in the tissues, a build up of carbon dioxide, and exercise, also increase the heart rate.

Nervous control of the blood vessels

The arteries are also regulated by the autonomic nervous system which responds to stress and relaxation, changes in blood pressure and in the chemical composition of the blood. The highest control comes from the cortex in the brain. This is the part that is concerned with intellectual and motor functions. There is a direct influence on the hypothalamus which is responsible for maintaining the internal environment of the whole body.

When stress stimulates the cortex, it sends signals to the hypothalamus to stimulate the sympathetic nervous system so that the body can either face or run away from the stress. This causes the body to dilate the blood vessels to the heart and muscles (so that they receive more oxygen) and contract the blood vessels to most other body parts. In this way we can run or fight, using our muscle power. More blood vessels are constricted than dilated, giving an overall net effect of vessels constriction. This increases the peripheral resistance of the body, raises the blood pressure and gives the heart more work to do. When the stress passes, the sympathetic stimulation decreases and the blood vessels relax and dilate.

The calibre of the arterioles depends on many things. The calibre constantly changes so that the amount of blood in the body can be evenly distributed through all the different areas. Some parts shut off supply for a while as others turn their supply on. Psychic and emotional factors, oxygen demand, time of day, food, mental or physical activity, buildup of waste products such as lactic acid and heat, all modify the flow.

When there is excessive stimulation of the sympathetic nervous system as can easily happen in the fast and stressful pace of modern city life, the vessels can become constricted for excessively long periods of time. Eventually the muscles governing constriction go into spasm. Thus the blood pressure stays at an elevated level, preventing oxygen and nutrients from reaching the organs of the body in sufficient quantity and permitting build up of potentially harmful waste material. The whole body becomes weakened and the individual suffers from exhaustion and hypertension.

Blood pressure

The blood is always under pressure. When the heart contracts during systole, the pressure rises. This is the maximum blood pressure called the *systolic blood pressure*. When the heart relaxes during the phase of diastole, the blood pressure is at its minimum, and is called *diastolic blood pressure*. The blood levels should be known to properly understand the state of physical health. Of the two pressures the diastolic is more important in cases of hypertension because it reflects the state of the autonomic nervous system and tone of the blood vessels. The systolic pressure reflects the state of the heart, and it is important in hypertensive people when the disease has involved the heart and caused it to fail.

The blood pressure is written so that the systolic pressure is said first and/or written on the top of the diastolic pressure. The normal blood pressure in a meat-eating, highly technological society is 120 over 80 millimetres of mercury pressure (mm Hg), written as 120/80 mm Hg. This is the average pressure only, and is calculated on the majority of the people in the community. It differs from individual to individual, and there is no one perfect pressure. Factors such as time of day, temperature, activity, stress, mental state, age, diet (vegetarian and non-vegetarian) and season, all affect the pressure and it varies from moment to moment in all of us. For example, the older you are, the greater the chance that your blood pressure will be higher than average. Children are usually within the range of 75–90 mm Hg, while the elderly are up to 130–150 mm Hg systolic. Obesity also tends to raise the blood pressure, while resting lowers it. It is important to take into account the sequence of blood pressure over a few days or weeks, especially from the doctor's point of view. It is difficult to judge from just one reading what exactly is going on within the body. It requires great skill to take the blood pressure reading accurately and to interpret what that reading means. Therefore, we do not recommend that you buy a sphygmomanometer in order to measure your own blood pressure. Most people who do so tend to make mistakes in reading it and in interpretation, causing themselves worry and suffering for no good reason. It is better to let the doctor do the work. He has the perspective of many years of experience in taking blood pressure readings.

Abnormal blood pressure

What is the dividing line between normality and abnormality? This is a question that most doctors have been arguing about for a long time. No exact definition can be given. For, the moment you define high blood pressure you are committed to a framework that does not permit much flexibility. Many people may be on the borderline of hypertension without having either symptoms or measurable signs of disease other than the fact that their blood pressure is a little higher than the pressure of the next person. If a rigid threshold is set, such a person may be bound to a drug regime for the rest of his life just in case he has hypertension.

The fact remains that no one knows what hypertension really is. Hypertension is the name given to a state of the body and mind characterized by a raised blood pressure. The arbitrary borderline accepted by most doctors as being the point to consider drug therapy or other means of lowering the blood pressure, is taken at 140–90 mm Hg. This is applied to younger people especially, while varying degrees of higher pressure are tolerated in older individuals. This is because in the young there is more chance of developing serious complications than in the elderly, and because the sign of increasing blood pressure in a younger person is a serious one, to be closely watched.

Hypertension

Hypertension in any of its many forms is a serious disease. Even a mild case with very few symptoms (subjective experience of disease) lowers the life span and decreases the quality of the remaining years.

The form of hypertension with which we are concerned here is called *essential hypertension,* accounting for approximately eighty percent of cases. This form has no known medical cause. The other twenty percent is caused by either medically or surgically identifiable causes. We suggest that you consult your doctor at the first signs of high blood pressure to determine if your case is essential or correctable hypertension. Essential hypertension is also reversible, but not by medical means alone. It is only through the combination and balance of medicine and yoga that the battle of high blood pressure can be won.

Hypertension is particularly dangerous as it is a 'silent' illness. Most people with high blood pressure show few or no symptoms of the disease for many years yet despite this, life-threatening consequences and complications can occur. The clinical course of hypertension is varied. It can be apparently slow and protracted or rapidly progressive and soon fatal.

In the mild form, the disease is usually complicated by one or more of the following: hardening of the arteries, disease of the blood vessels in the brain leading to rupture (a stroke, or cerebrovascular accident), heart attacks (myocardial infarction), kidney disease, stretching of the aorta (aneurysm), and disease of the small blood vessels at the periphery of the body, causing tissue destruction.

In the severe form, the kidneys are profoundly affected and eventually fail to function, leading to death within months or even weeks.

In both mild and severe cases the arterioles are constricted, increasing the peripheral resistance. The blood pressure maintains high levels, body organs are damaged and fail in their respective functions.

Actually hypertension is not a disease in itself, but a sign that there are underlying problems in the management of the internal environment and balance of the body at the physical, emotional and mental levels. Medicine has coined the term hypertension and this is exactly what the disease is, excessive tension in the body. It is tension of the whole body/ mind complex, resulting in imbalance of the nervous system. Coordination of bodily functions is impaired and all systems, including the cardiovascular system, suffer as a consequence. Those individuals who are predisposed to trouble due to weakness in this system, manifest disease on the physical plane. No doubt, if we look closely at the whole individual we shall see that there are problems at a deeper level as well.

Modern medicine has now realized that the mind plays at least some role in about 80 percent of disease, classifying this type of disease as psychosomatic, meaning 'of mind and body'. However, allopathy has yet to discover the full implications of this insight, and is still seeking to clarify the role of the psyche in physical illness. The yogic comprehension of the role of the mind in psychosomatic disease is practically expressed in techniques designed to remove psychological stress and its bodily effects. This is achieved through meditation, asana (physical postures), pranayama (breathing exercises) and other means that will have important implications in the treatments of the future.

The knowledge of yoga is especially relevant to high blood pressure as both heart and blood vessels respond very

18

readily to fluctuations in the mind and emotions. An unstable mind leads to an unstable body, and mental or emotional disturbance reflects into the cardiovascular system producing various symptoms, including an increase in blood pressure.

What is hypertension?

Before we can understand what causes high blood pressure we must understand what it is. Increased blood pressure results from the damming up of blood behind constricted arterioles, upsetting the balance of the heart and its vessels. Blood leaving the heart on its way to the cells of the body meets with excessive resistance, and the heart is therefore required to work harder to pump the blood through the narrowed vessels.

During times of rest the heart does not strain excessively because it does not have to deliver as much oxygen to the cells as it does during stress and exercise. However, the moment stress is placed upon the body, whether this be physical or mental, the oxygen demand increases and so does the work of the heart. When this happens over an extended period of time, the heart becomes permanently strained and eventually does not function properly. This leads to serious and even lethal complications.

In hypertension the body cannot adapt to the needs of its internal and external environment. When arterioles have remained in a constricted state for a period of time, the muscles around them spasm. The blood cannot supply oxygen needs and at the same time it cannot pick up the waste material produced, resulting in fatigue and exhaustion. It takes a great deal of rest to undo the damage caused by this spasm. Recent scientific research has proved that the sort of rest required cannot be gained even through sleep, but only through meditation.

Lactic acid is a chemical by-product of stress, manu-factured in muscle tissue when the oxygen supply does not keep up with the work output and its oxygen need. This is not a healthy state, and lactic acid must be eliminated during periods of rest, notably during sleep. Physiological monitoring during meditation shows that there is a decrease in the activity of the sympathetic nervous system, relaxing constriction of the blood vessels. This leads to an immediate drop in blood pressure and increases blood flow to the muscles supplying needed oxygen and removing lactic acid. Researchers Wallace and Benson have shown that during meditation the level of lactic acid in the body decreases four times faster than during normal activity and three times faster than during sleep.[1] This indicates that meditation is more efficient in repairing physical damage associated with hypertension.

Millions of years ago when our animal ancestors had to survive in a hostile environment the sympathetic system was a lifesaver. This system is concerned with the stress response mechanism as explained by the scientist Hans Selye. He showed that there are three basic components of the stress mechanism:

1. Alarm is registered by the sympathetic nervous system which triggers the adrenal glands to release adrenaline, and the pituitary gland to release other hormones.
2. The second stage is continuation of neural and endocrine reactions until the stressful situation has passed.
3. The third stage is one of exhaustion as the human organism requires rest to restore balance to the body. If there is no rest the stress hormones and reactions accumulate and destroy the body.

This stress reflex is still activated by the body and mind in stressful situations. It is a basic instinctual response seated deep within the oldest parts of our nervous system. Although it was essential to our ancestors' survival in the early days of man's evolution, it is less so today. In fact it is often out of control and has become more destructive than useful. This reaction is the basis of much of the disease we suffer today, in the form of psychosomatic and stress-related illness.

In some situations the stress reaction is necessary, but it is also something that must be properly controlled if it is to retain its usefulness to man and his society. For example, it is physiologically acceptable for the stress reaction to operate when our lives are being threatened, but if it operates when we are caught in a traffic jam or if we are late for work, then it serves no useful purpose. In the first situation the reaction powers our muscles and allows us to run or fight. In the second situation it triggers all the hormones and neurone circuits but the energy liberated is not utilized. The hormones build up and create toxins and poisons which exhaust the body. Simultaneously the sympathetic nervous system shuts down capillary beds and prevents enough oxygen getting to tissues. This is associated with a feeling of frustration, tension, anxiety and loss of mental clarity. There is an overall decrease in body efficiency rather than an increase.

The normal and non-neurotic way to handle stressful situations such as traffic jams and being late for work is to accept the situation as it is, in a relaxed and positive frame of mind. This occurs if we are aware that nothing can be achieved by undue worry. Survival and happiness today require that we tune into the overall situation involving ourselves, the people around us, and the total environment of the here and now. Perceptiveness, wisdom and oneness are the ingredients for effective action and survival in today's world. We must raise our consciousness above the animal-instinctual and become more truly human. This involves increased awareness of our own inner workings and greater control over ourselves.

A meditative attitude towards the world allows us to control the adrenaline release and the sympathetic over-stimulation that accompanies most kinds of stressful situations. This is achieved through increased understanding of the inner workings of mind and brain, which is enhanced through meditation. When the mind becomes more relaxed it tends to view stressful situations in a completely different light. Instead of becoming frustrated by the little things of life, wider spaces are opened up to our view, and an inner world emerges that has as much, if not more, importance than the outer world. This is the world of intuition (inner knowledge and understanding) and by tuning in to this world of intuition we can prevent disease and remove hypertension from our lives.

Do you have hypertension?

Many people have elevated blood pressure without knowing it. For the majority, hypertension is not firmly established but becomes noticeable through its symptoms. Then, when the stress or emotional tension is removed for a while, the blood pressure drops. This is called labile hypertension and is thought to be the precursor of essential hypertension.

Hypertension is caused by the stresses and strains of modern living. If you are in any way subject to these stresses and feel they are affecting you, then you have a chance of getting hypertension. Whether or not this actually occurs depends on your own constitution; whether you are predisposed to suffering increased blood pressure, ulcers, or some other form of disease. Everyone has his or her own weak point.

To know whether you have hypertension or not, you must ask yourself the same questions a doctor might ask if he were examining you for high blood pressure. This is called taking a medical history. The doctor then conducts a full physical examination and, if required, may carry out some laboratory procedures. These questions would be foremost in his mind:

How long ago was your last physical examination?

In this way the doctor can check up and compare what your blood pressure was last time it was taken and see if there has been any significant change.

Is there a family history of hypertension?

If other members of your family or close relatives have had hypertension, then it is more likely that you will also suffer from the same type of condition.

22

Have you ever had kidney trouble, protein in your urine or any type of urinary disturbance?

Kidney disease is one of the treatable and reversible causes of high blood pressure, and must be eliminated from a list of possible causes before starting treatment for essential hypertension.

Have you had any of the following symptoms that could imply hypertension?

These are: headaches at the back of the head, especially in the morning; palpitations which are sudden and quite perceptible, increased speed of the heart, like a thumping in the chest; nervousness; dizziness; light-headedness; lassitude; apathy; depression; anxiety; uncomfortable feelings inside that cannot be explained; increased irritability; emotional upset.

Have you had any of the following symptoms that could suggest a more serious degree of hypertension?

They are: headache, breathlessness, palpitations, languor, feeling of fullness in the head, disturbance of vision, sleeplessness, flushed complexion, loss of appetite, decreased memory and concentration, nausea (a feeling of wanting to vomit), spinning feelings.

Do you have any evidence of heart disease, kidney disease, thyroid disease, or adrenal overactivity?

These can only be answered by a competent doctor. If you can answer yes to *any* of the above then you should contact a doctor and a competent yoga teacher who can help you to remove such troubling symptoms. If you feel even slightly unwell it is the first sign of some inner disturbance which could lead on to more serious disease. Therefore, you should take such signs seriously and do something constructive about removing them. The most positive step you can make is to start to practise yoga, as this will not only remove symptoms but also prevent further disease.

You should be aware too, of the possibility of being a potential candidate for high blood pressure if you lead a hectic life full of worries and concerns that often make you feel tense and unhappy. If you feel unhappy about any aspect of life then this is the potential start for future disease.

Profile

Though many people of varied types and personality suffer from high blood pressure there is one type of person who is by far in the majority – the young or middle-aged business-man. Friedman and Rosenman, both heart specialists and dealing particularly with the cardiovascular system, state that in their medical practice (reflecting the American situation) they found typical cardiac patients had in common a competitive, aggressive, ambitious, stressful lifestyle.[2] They demonstrated that almost all their patients were ambitious career men. This, however, should be kept in perspective. Most of the 700,000 Americans who died from high blood pressure in 1976 were businessmen in the middle of vigorous careers. In the same year it was estimated that 24 million Americans suffered from hypertension, and the number is steadily growing. Due to increasing numbers of hypertensive patients, doctors are adding the term 'hypertensive epidemic' to their vocabulary.

If the above description fits you then you should take note and be warned of the possibilities. The best solution for those people who are not prepared to give up their lifestyle because of the threat of disease (which will put an end to their lifestyle anyway) is that they should take up yoga and meditation. In this way they will minimize the harmful effects of stress and can live more relaxed and fuller lives.

Possible consequences

The main danger of having hypertension is not the fact that the blood pressure itself is raised, but the harmful con-sequences of raised blood pressure. There are many things which can go wrong as the blood vessels feed into every

24

organ of the body. When they are constricted, preventing the inflow of blood and thus the distribution of oxygen and removal of wastes, tissue damage occurs. This prevents the organs from functioning. In the case of the brain, heart, kidneys, etc., this is lethal. Some manifestations are:

- *Heart disease*: The heart, as it becomes more and more strained, increases in size, damaging its internal components such as the valves, and thus impairing total function. The heart also becomes more prone to heart attack (death of part of a muscle) as high blood pressure is associated with hardening of the arteries.
- *The brain*: Oxygen supply to the brain is reduced so that it cannot function at optimum level. At first this may result in headaches, dizziness and a feeling of the world spinning (vertigo). Later, emotional imbalance and deterioration of concentration and memory occur followed by more serious complications of organic brain deterioration (encephalopathy), rupture of arteries (stroke) leading to paralysis and death.
- *The eyes*: Blurring of the vision, and sudden, progressive loss of vision may result. There can also be doubling of the vision (diplopia) or other defects.
- *Kidneys*: Dysfunction occurs which may result in the inability to produce urine. This allows the toxins of the body to build up and death can result.
- *Malignant hypertension*: A serious form of the disease. The blood pressure may rise to astronomical heights and death approaches rapidly.

The consequences of hypertension are unpleasant. Knowing the possibilities can help you to find a successful method of cure. One can avoid these complications before they start by applying yoga to the present regime of treatment. By relaxing body and mind, yoga allows the blood vessels to relax, ensuring a good supply of blood, oxygen and nutrition to the tissues. This, enhanced by the increased flow of prana, will feed the tissues and aid in the process of regeneration and rejuvenation.

25

The Medical View

The patterns of living in society contribute to good or poor health, and the cause of high blood pressure, or any disease, involves many aspects of our lives. Hypertension is a good example of modern social disease.

Hypertension has several specific causes. It appears that a combination of these is responsible for the increased incidence in high blood pressure over the last decade. These causes include heredity, age, smoking, high fat diet, sedentary lifestyle, personality, temperament and emotions.

Heredity

If both your parents have hypertension the chances of you also becoming hypertensive are forty-five percent higher than normal. If one parent was hypertensive your chances are thirty percent higher than normal. Thus, the influence of heredity does play a part in the causation of hypertension by laying down the basic characteristics which will be modified by the environment and learned patterns of behaviour. While some of these factors may be inherited, many are simply the result of parental attitude. *All are reversible.*

Age

The peak incidence of hypertension falls in the forty to sixty years age group, though the number of young people with hypertension is on the increase.

26

With advancing age there is a normal increase in blood pressure in most people, short of the range of hypertension. However, with the advance of time there is a greater chance of building up the various aggravating factors which lead to hypertension. Eventually those people whose circulatory system is susceptible and whose lifestyle is also conducive to illness, cross that threshold which is the vague zone between normal and high blood pressure.

It is obvious that ageing and subsequent deterioration of the physical body facilitate the disease process. At the same time, buildup of toxins, stress hormones and tension hasten ageing. A degenerative disease, such as hypertension, manifests more in adults and very rarely in children. With advancing age, there is also a greater chance of hardening of the arteries, with its accompanying increased blood pressure.

Smoking

There is now incontrovertible evidence that smoking is harmful to the health. It is known that as well as the increased chance of lung cancer and lung disease in general, smoking contributes to hardening of the blood vessels of the heart (ischaemic heart disease); deterioration of the peripheral vessels (peripheral vascular disease) leading to greater peripheral resistance; and to inflammation of the optic nerve (optic neuritis). It has been observed that all these diseases are more common in smokers than in non-smokers.

Cholesterol and high fat diet

Cholesterol and increased blood fats (lipids) have been correlated with an increased incidence of blood vessel disorder. When vessels are diseased there is a greater chance of developing high blood pressure. A diet excessively rich in fats is unhealthy. Therefore, even with normal blood pressure one should limit the intake of fatty foods in order to maintain maximum health. High blood pressure plus excessive dietary fat is thought to hasten the process of deposition of fat on the vessel walls, and speeds hardening of the arteries.

27

Sedentary lifestyle

The mechanization of civilization and emphasis on city life has led to a decrease in the proportion of people who take vigorous exercise. Technological advancement has led to the widespread use of motor vehicles, cinema, television, books and all mechanical appliances. There is less physical activity required around the home, office and in recreation. Items that were once considered a luxury are now viewed in terms of necessity. This is all part of 'progress.'

The proportion of sedentary workers and business executives, who are most prone to hypertension, has increased. This has been paralleled by a massive increase in the number of people with high blood pressure. Statistics and experiments have proved that inadequate physical exercise weakens the body, leaving it prone to high blood pressure, especially when it is associated with mental stress.

Personality, stress and emotions

Research by psychiatrist Thomas Holmes has led other researchers to believe that constant stress, whether mental or emotional, weakens bodily resistance to disease. In one study Holmes and his colleague, Richard Rahe, found that over seventy-nine percent of those people who had undergone major life changes, such as taking a new job, divorce, death in the family, developed some kind of illness within two years of the change. Only thirty-seven percent who experienced minor life changes developed such illnesses.

Investigators have used emotional stress to trigger high blood pressure in experimental animals for over thirty years.

It was suggested that emotional arousal leads to high blood pressure via the sympathetic nervous system and cell metabolism. Changes in metabolism may alter the structure of the blood vessels, increasing their resistance to flow.

In their study of the increased incidence of heart disease, cardiologists Meyer Friedman and R.H. Rosenman turned from such factors as diet, exercise and blood type to personality and work-related factors.[3] They changed their

28

approach when an upholsterer who was refurnishing their waiting room remarked that the chairs were only worn on the front edge. The two workers consistently found that almost all of their cardiac patients had in common a competitive, aggressive, ambitious, stressful lifestyle. They demonstrated that career men, climbing the prestige ladder at a breakneck pace, have a higher level of fat in the bloodstream, excreting larger quantities of stress hormones, indicating that these hormones are produced in excess. They called this group Type A personality and found they were more prone to heart attacks than Type B, who are more easygoing people. Friedman and Rosenman suggest that Type A people can alter their personalities and reduce the chance of heart disease if they become more open and relaxed.

The classical viewpoint held by many psychologists and psychiatrists of the role of personality in essential hypertension is one associated with a picture of external friendliness and self-control beneath which there are strong aggressions and anxiety. Anxiety is intensified by the patient's fears of expressing his aggression, and a constant conflict ensues.

We react to internal emotional and mental stress, and to environmental situations, according to the nature of our personality. This is a subjective phenomenon. That is, the effect of the external or internal stimulus depends on the way in which we interpret it. Anything or any circumstance can be stress-provoking, depending on our attitude towards it. Even sport or recreational activity can provoke a negative response in our inner being. If we are internally strong we handle the situation in a mature manner and solve the problems causing stress. A negative view, from the negative side of our personality, creates tension. If we get caught up in this it feeds on our energy, weakens us and creates disease.

Cause

It has been shown that eighty percent of cases of hypertension have no known medical cause and these are known as *essential* or *idiopathic* hypertension.

There is controversy concerning the nature of essential hypertension. According to one scientific theory it is considered to be a specific disease. Another theory maintains that high blood pressure is a graded characteristic of the population, like height or weight. There are many theories, and each reflects the fact that medical science does not fully understand this disease. There are obviously various factors yet to be uncovered and perhaps some priorities must be reversed. To understand the whole disease requires evaluation of all factors. When we add up all the known and uncertain possible causes, we begin to pierce the veil of the idiopathic hypertensive. That is, the term idiopathic reflects the uncertainty in the minds of medical practitioners and researchers as to the exact cause of high blood pressure. When the whole picture is understood, the word 'idiopathic' will no longer be necessary.

The factors discussed in this chapter are those recognized by medical science to play a part in high blood pressure on the basis of experimental evidence. Five of the six factors listed pertain purely to the physical body. It is obvious, therefore, that medical science regards the physical factors as being the most important. However, there are certain missing links in the chain of doctors' understanding, and most will freely admit this. A new approach to cause and treatment is required.

Treatment

There is no specific treatment for essential hypertension because medical science has found no specific cause for this disorder. The aim of therapy is to lower the blood pressure using rest, diet, avoidance of stress and drugs.

General medical advice: Counselling on how to live a healthy life includes diet management to reduce the intake of fats and salts in order to lower the pressure and reduce the chance of hardening the arteries. Obesity is reduced by diet. Smoking is stopped and emotional stress avoided. Exercise within the range of tolerance is recommended.

Antihypertensive drugs: Once you start on drug therapy you must take these drugs for the rest of your life. In most cases drugs lower the blood pressure without undue side effects. However, you must continue medication even when the symptoms are ameliorated and, at the surface, hypertension is cured. If you stop drug therapy you risk your blood pressure shooting up to its original level or higher, with unpleasant effects. This is known as the rebound phenomenon. It occurs because drugs do not remove the root cause of hypertension, but only suppress it. Drugs can also cause unpleasant side effects. Only yoga gets to the root cause of the disease in a safe, efficient manner. However, drugs can effectively reduce a dangerously high blood pressure as a prelude to more long-range yogic therapy, and can then be withdrawn.

Thus, medical therapy rests on drugs and general advice. At the same time the aware and concerned physician acquaints himself with his patient's personal and family problems in order to relieve them and to reduce tension which may be aggravating the patient's internal state.

Good communication between doctor and patient, and trust and faith on both sides, ensure better management and a greater chance of successful cure.

Prognosis (long-term outlook)

The picture painted by modern medical science is not a pretty one. It is known that hypertension is a life-threatening disease. Also, once you start on drugs, unless you practise yoga, you are going to be dependent on those drugs for the rest of your life. From our experience with yoga students who have benefited from yoga techniques, we know that the use of yoga can not only remove symptoms as do drugs, but it also strikes at the root of hypertension by remoulding both mind and body. Yoga has always been available but until recently the medical profession has not had access to it. Now, scientific data has come to light and proved that yoga can replace drugs in the treatment of hypertension.

31

The Yogic View

According to yoga the mind is the most important component in the cause of hypertension. It is the common denominator underlying all the aspects considered by medical science. The medical list of causes is correct. However, fuller and deeper understanding of the cause of hypertension requires that the list be expanded and the priorities rearranged. You should note that the word 'idiopathic' is not included in the yogic terminology.

Yoga's classification, therefore, is as follows:

1. *Mental cause*: The core or essence of hypertensive disease is in the mind.
2. *Pranic cause*: Hypertension is also associated with disturbance in the energy systems of the body.
3. *Stress in the personality*: These factors are determined by mind and should come under 'mental cause' but are classified separately for clarity.
4. *Physical causes*: This aspect includes five of the six medical causes, most important of which are:
   a) lifestyle: modern living, sleeping habits, smoking, diet and sedentary occupation
   b) heredity
   c) age and ageing.

Yoga therefore agrees with medicine, but through experience and a deeper understanding of the whole human organism sees that the mind plays an important role in the functioning of the body. It can maintain and enhance health or cause disease such as hypertension. The physical aspect plays a minor part in the causation mechanism of hypertension.

Modern medical science also attributes importance to the mental aspects. Recent research points to the significance of mental tension and personality factors. However, this research has yet to be fully integrated into medical thought before its practical application. It is this field that yoga can aid most. It offers explanations of cause and a working model of mind in relation to the other dimensions of the human being. Practical techniques are designed to remove mental tension, layer by layer, until tension-free and joyful existence is experienced, free from the curse of hypertension.

The mind and body are one. They are not merely linked but are interlocked and reflect each other. What we are seeing on the physical plane as hypertension is reflected from the mental levels into the brain and into the body.

In the fifteenth chapter of the *Bhagavad Gita* it is said that the roots of an imperishable tree are at the top and the branches are below. Today science is verifying this. Medical science has dissected the physical body and found the topsy-turvy tree mentioned in the *Gita* to be the brain and spinal column. The trunk is the spinal cord, the branches are the peripheral nerves winding their way through the body, and the roots are the brain sunk into the soil of the mind.

The body is directly influenced by the mind. If a positive attitude as well as strength and health of mind is maintained, then the body is well nourished and flourishes. If there are mental problems, neuroses, negativity, deep-rooted complexes and mental tensions, the tree withers and illnesses such as hypertension appear as signs that something is not functioning correctly. This indicates that work must be done on the body and mind or death will eventuate.

The five bodies

The yoga shastras (ancient texts) deal with the mind in its proper perspective. When we, too, gain this perspective we can deal with the mind and hypertension as easily and effectively as the yogis who wrote the ancient texts. They saw that our being has five components, or *koshas* (sheaths).

The physical body has two parts: *annamaya kosha*, the actual physical body, and *pranamaya kosha*, the vital energy sheath, also called the bioplasmic or bioenergy body by scientists who appear to have photographed its reflection in an electric field (Kirlian photography). It provides a subtle framework that organizes the physical body and supplies energy for the movement and metabolism of parts.

The mind has two parts: *manomaya kosha*, the lower mind sheath, is concerned with intellectual and rational activity and is much more subtle that the physical body. *Vijnanamaya kosha*, the higher mind sheath, is more subtle still. It is concerned with intuition, inspirational and creative thought and action and it contacts the spiritual realm.

There is a fifth and still more subtle body called *anandamaya kosha*, the causal or bliss body. This is a body of light. The five bodies surround the *jivatma*, or individual soul.

Each of the bodies must be nourished by proper lifestyle and food. For the physical body, moderation is required in diet, sleep and general lifestyle, to prevent hypertension. The mind must maintain balance with the physical body and be kept free of anxiety and stress. Each component of the whole is dependent on every other component for its maintenance and effective functioning. We can imagine the relation of mind to body in the following example: When we make bread we mix flour and water and add a few more essential ingredients. If we imagine the flour to be the body and the water to be the mind then the dough represents the living being. In order for the dough to be edible and thereby serve and fulfil its function, it must receive fire and air and bake at the right temperature for just the right time. If we live the normal, hassled, stressful existence without some means of coping with stress, then we are sure to either undercook or burn the bread. Yoga is the means to ensure that the bread of life is properly cooked and life-giving.

34

Mental Cause

Every person has some neurotic tendencies or mental problems which cause periods of unhappiness, tension, depression, anxiety to one degree or another. Very few people are totally free from these influences. We can see the results of our personal problems and negative tendencies in our health and environment. Mental weaknesses cause ill health, difficult interpersonal relationships and have even wider ramifications as seen, for example, in a disordered and polluted environment. Of course, there is the positive side of our nature and we should not forget this. However, to become more positive and remove the cause of hypertension, at the same time preventing future disease, we must become more aware of what is actually causing this disease. We must see how it has come about, and remove it.

When we are subjected to a polluted atmosphere and the fast pace of modern society, mental, emotional and physical tensions build up. The mind is a more subtle component than the physical and subject to faster change. It is impressed, or indented, by our internal reaction to external events, and this causes mental patterns to form. The habit patterns can be conducive to good or poor health. The body, being more gross and less flexible than the mind, takes longer to change. However, change does occur. If we allow tensions to build up within the mind through lack of awareness, these first cause us mental problems such as depression, anxiety and fear,

35

and thus we suffer. Eventually, these processes of the mind wear down the body like the stormy sea battering cliffs and coves. Thus changes occur.

Mental tensions filter into the physical via the pranic structure. They first gain access via the brain, which is the gateway between mind and body. The brain is part of the physical body though it is intimately linked with the mental body. The brain is the crossroads between the inner and outer world, the junction of individuality, enabling us to communicate our inner individual experiences to the outside world and to react to external happenings from moment to moment. It is our controlling instrument for external communication and self-expression. If it is kept in good condition, the quality of our lives is then greatly enhanced.

The brain controls the autonomic nervous system which regulates the blood pressure. When it is imbalanced due to higher and more subtle disturbances, we get hypertension through excessive sympathetic stimulation. The brain also affects our lifestyle and environment.

There has been a great deal of research into the mind with the establishment of a new branch of science, para-psychology. This science seeks to investigate the effects of the mind on the body and to discover the basis of certain paranormal experiences such as telepathy, psychokinesis, psychotronics, faith healing, etc.

In America, the Academy of Parapsychology and Medicine has been set up and is investigating, among other fields, unorthodox healing systems such as psychic healing, radionics, acupuncture and yoga. Their work and the efforts of other researchers is outlining 'maps of consciousness', maps of the mind, charting the effects of mind on body. Through this research more will be gleaned about psychosomatic diseases, of which hypertension is one, as well as the role of mind in all illnesses.

Dr Elmer Green, head of the Psychophysiology Laboratory in the Research Department at the Menninger Foundation, states that as many as eighty percent of diseases

36

have a psychosomatic component in their cause. He bases this view on his work with biofeedback. Biofeedback is teaching people to directly control their so-called 'involuntary' functions of the body by using machines to monitor internal changes in body systems. These machines then relay this information to the practitioner, making him aware of subtle alterations in his body that are normally not perceptible. For instance, hypertensive patients are now learning to regulate the calibre of the blood vessels in response to a flashing light that tells them if the vessels are too wide or too narrow. Biofeedback makes it *clear*, beyond doubt, that the mind has the power to change body functions by directing energy from the pranic body.

When we say psychosomatic disease we mean diseases caused by the unbalancing and disorganization of mental processes, which proceed as though they were disconnected from our control. The brain normally programs the body by sending excitatory or inhibitory impulses to certain areas, and by regulating balance of the autonomic and sensory-motor components of the nervous system. When disorder and chaos occur in the higher realms, the brain circuits are altered and cells of the brain, *neurones*, are disconnected and reconnected to new locations which have maladaptive and destructive effects on the rest of the body. Irregularities of the blood pressure regulation system are caused in this way. The mind works through the individual patterns of the body and our energy flows according to the channels opened and closed to it. Heredity and lifestyle largely determine the channels for mental energy by developing habits and patterns of living which affect the circuits in the brain and create channels of least resistance for the energy to flow through.

Levels of mind

In psychosomatic disease we find the whole mind affecting the body. The mind has breadth, width and depth. The individual mind is but a drop in the infinite ocean of the cosmic mind. The individual mind may only be a drop, but

37

from our perspective it is a huge drop and is not at all well understood by most cultures today.

Modern psychology has divided the mind into three basic units: the conscious aspects, the subconscious and the unconscious. The conscious part is only the tip of the iceberg which is the mind. The subconscious and unconscious form the greater, hidden part. There are other terms but these three are the main ones. More recent psychological growth has founded a new branch of the tree called transpersonal psychology, which deals more with the relation of individual minds in the ocean of cosmic mind.

In real terms it does not matter into how many levels you divide the mind, for they all affect each other. Hypertension is caused by all the levels of the mind interacting with each other. The conscious, or gross part of the mind, knows that we have hypertension. We are aware of changes in our body in the form of disease symptoms which alert us to the fact that we may have hypertension.

The subconscious is a subtle area, the vague zone just beneath the surface of consciousness, presenting an interface between conscious and unconscious. For most of us it is just a blurry impression. However, in meditation it becomes an area as distinct as the conscious, and you can dive into it and experience it with your awareness as you would this normal waking consciousness.

The unconscious is the sublime or causal area of tremendous power reserve. If the subconscious were not present as a buffer or wall against the force of the unconscious, then this energy would come rushing up into consciousness and flood our awareness with feelings which we could not handle. The unconscious contains the archetypes of our being, the vast energies and powers which have taken form as the most basic drives and instincts of our lives. For example, the archetypes of the mother and father exist at the very depths of our being. When in this life we experience negative feelings towards our parents we find conflict occurring between the archetypal ideal and the actuality. This conflict may be suppressed, that is, the energy may be pushed back into the unconscious areas of the mind. Yet it still exerts an influence over our lives, without our being aware of it. It is these complex interactions of energy that create neuroses and mental suffering.

The unconscious forces next reflect into the subconscious mind which reflects into the body functions. Only one tenth of the mind and brain are consciously utilized. The rest is dormant, subconscious, and controls the autonomic functions of heart rate, breathing, blood vessel regulation and so on. If you are predisposed to imbalance of the blood pressure regulating mechanism, then the negative energy manifests in the physical body through this weak point and causes increased peripheral resistance.

Hypertension is a result of the accumulated sense impressions, thoughts, fears, joys, memories, ideas, knowledge, and anxieties that are stored in the deeper levels of mind. If the negative side overwhelms the positive, then the energy released surges out of the subconscious and affects those areas of the brain that are regulated by the subconscious mind. This occurs before we become conscious of the fact that we have hypertension, and the process takes some time before it fully manifests in the physical body as disease.

Mind and lifestyle

Mind is the basis of hypertension for it controls our personality, emotions, lifestyle and habits. Aspects of lifestyle such as smoking, high fat diet, heredity and ageing all come under the influence of mind as it is the more subtle and powerful aspect of our being. Mind gives the objective reality our subjective interpretation. This aspect of life is unique to man. He is the only living creature who can shape his environment to suit his desires and abilities. He can change his own life and thereby affect the world around in a positive or negative way. If positive, he remains healthy and fulfils his life, but if negative, man creates for himself conditions conducive to the development of high blood pressure.

The Pranic Cause

When the mind becomes tense, the ramifications spread throughout the whole body, changing structure and function, and affecting us in many gross and subtle ways. Because the mind affects the body via the pranic body, the first change caused by mental tension occurs in the pranic body which interpenetrates and vitalizes the physical sheath. Thoughts produced by the mind are charged with energy, the force of which works on the body. Mental energy (chitta) and physical vitality (prana), are both intimately connected.

In the physical body we can see the effects of thoughts redirecting energy when we take the example of the anxious person developing diarrhoea, rapid pulse and faster breathing, or the depressed person who develops constipation and slower movements. Thus the energy or prana of the body depends on the mind for its direction, but when there are mental problems and neuroses the energy is not directed properly into the lower bodies. This changes the structure of the pranic and physical bodies, and those areas which are the weakest suffer most from this imbalance. In the case of the hypertensive, the blood vessel system is affected.

The pranic body

Yoga understands prana as the energy responsible for all the vital functions of digestion, respiration, excretion, transmission of nervous impulses, circulation of blood and

40

so on. It is divided into five specific kinds, according to location and function.

Apana throws out impurities and creates strength. It is associated with the earth element and therefore moves downward, acting below the navel so that it expels water from the kidneys, faeces, semen and the foetus from the womb.

Samana extends from the diaphragm to the navel and is linked with the water element. It causes secretion of the digestive juices in the digestive tract and aids the kidneys, spleen and urinary process. It distributes food to the blood to nourish the heart, brain and body.

Prana is associated with the fire element and draws vitality from the food and air. It is part of the total body energy, also called prana, and controls the energy from the diaphragm to the mouth. Therefore, prana is associated with breath and heart. When most people speak of prana they are speaking of the total body prana but associate it with this specific manifestation of the total prana. Prana moves upward and aids in the production of sound as well as moving food to the stomach, creating sweat, maintaining body heat, oxygenating and circulating the blood, and causing hunger and thirst.

Udana is the aspect of prana that lifts the body up and keeps it from falling. It also controls vomiting. It is associated with the air element and aids in production of sound and singing. Its body area is from the throat to the cerebellum.

Vyana is the aspect of prana which pervades the entire body, coordinating all the body functions and the five pranas. It helps sensory nerves, beating of the heart, blood circulation and faculties which extend throughout the body, such as blood, nerves and lymph. It also works in the minor divisions of prana in the eyes, mouth, nose and eyelids and in the function of yawning, sneezing, belching and hiccoughing.

These are the five interlinked and interdependent aspects of the pranamaya kosha or pranic body. Imbalance in any one, especially vyana or samana, makes the body especially prone to hypertension, circulatory defects and neuro-circulatory imbalance.

41

Nadis

Prana and chitta are circulated through a network of flow-ways called nadis. There are 72,000 nadis or energy channels in the body. They are organized in much the same pattern as the blood vessels, for they have three main channels of flow: *ida* (the mental channel), *pingala* (the vital channel) and *sushumna* (the spiritual channel). These branch and subdivide into finer and finer channels permeating every atom of the body. The nadis compose an energizing infrastructure within every cell, tissue and organ of the physical body. Any blockage or impurity in the nadis leads to disease. Blockages are due to chaotic thought patterns or stressful lifestyle.

Through its network of nadis, the pranic body acts as a lattice for blood vessels to build upon. In hypertension this lattice gradually weakens the blood vessels. This is caused by an imbalance in the mind, acting via the brain and hypothalamus to initiate excess sympathetic activity and increased peripheral resistance.

On the physical level, the arteries which are the active dynamic component of the circulatory system reflect pingala nadi, whereas the veins, which are the passive receptive component, reflect ida nadi. Sushumna nadi, which lies in the centre of the spinal cord, is mirrored in the vast capillary network which extends throughout the whole body.

Hypertension is the result of an imbalance in the nadis in which pingala becomes predominant. Pingala is associated with heat, the colour red, extroversion and dynamism. Hypertension is linked to the pingala nadi because the arterial tree which branches out from the heart is most dynamic. The blood it carries is red because of its high oxygen content.

This disease is also associated with extroversion, ambition and wanting to get ahead in the world. There is the tendency for the mind to become involved in the sensual side to the exclusion of the internal side of man. There is nothing wrong with the sensual aspect of existence, but it must be balanced by an inner view as well, thus attaining a middle path – the path of sushumna, balance in all things.

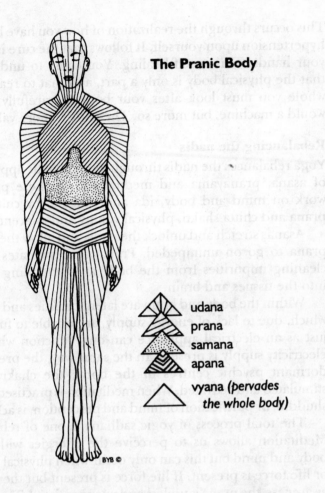

The Pranic Body

udana
prana
samana
apana
vyana (pervades
the whole body)

BYB ©

When pingala becomes dominant the sympathetic system functions in excess, resulting in hypertension and other stress related diseases. In this way the pranic system reflects into the mind and body.

You must become aware of the pranic body so that the physical body can be viewed in correct perspective. Awareness is gained through yoga, and is in itself a healing factor, for when awareness is attained one automatically adjusts the lifestyle and thought processes so that health is increased.

This occurs through the realization of how you have brought hypertension upon yourself. It follows that the cure is also in your hands. This is self-healing. You come to understand that the physical body is only a part, and that to realize the whole you must look after your body as carefully as you would a machine, but more so. The body is more valuable.

Rebalancing the nadis

Yoga rebalances the nadis through its systematic application of asana, pranayama and meditation. All these practices work on mind and body, ida and pingala, by cultivating prana and chitta shakti, physical vitality and awareness.

Asanas stretch and unlock the nadis and allow the flow of prana to go on unimpeded. Pranayama circulates prana, cleaning impurities from the body and extending vitality into the tissues and brain.

Within the body and brain are latent faculties and powers which, due to lack of energy supply, are unable to function, just as an electrical appliance can only function when the electricity supply is present. In the same way, the previously dormant psychic centres of the body, the chakras, are stimulated and activated. When meditation is practised, chitta shuddhi, or purification of mind and perception, is achieved.

The total process of yogic sadhana is one of rebalance. Meditation allows us to perceive the energies within the body and mind but this can only occur when physical energy or life force is present. If life force is present but there is no awareness, the prana is useless and unappreciated. Therefore, both prana and chitta must be present in order to achieve balance and integration, true relaxation of tension and the joyful experience (ida) of glowing health (pingala). Hypertension vanishes, just as a soap bubble does when pricked.

When the forces of mind and body are in balanced harmony, having been purified and strengthened, sushumna nadi and its dynamic form of spiritual awareness, full of peace, light and knowledge, can blossom, transforming and adding a new hyperaware dimension to our existence.

44

Stress and the Personality

There is no doubt that personality plays an important role in the development of certain kinds of diseases, for personality determines our ability to handle stress. Stress is not an objective entity. It is a subjective reaction to an external or internal situation. Any situation can produce stress even if it is designed to bring relaxation, like playing golf or going swimming. It all depends on our personal view of the situation. The way in which we react is determined by past experience and our type of personality.

The endocrine and nervous systems are linked with, and respond directly to, the brain and the mind. Both affect personality, which is built up through our past experiences. Personality determines action and creates channels or grooves called habits. These lead us in to a seemingly endless maze of actions and thoughts. You can change this situation for the better by changing your brain patterns, personality and habits. Thus you free yourself of all restricting influences and experience life unhindered by past memories and future worry. This is spontaneous creativity.

Medical science has classified two basic types of people – stable and labile.

Stable people are more independent, with greater motor control, greater resistance to noise and sensory deprivation, have higher mental health on psychological testing, and are less susceptible to conditioning.

45

The *labile* personality is the precursor of psychosomatic disease and mental illness. People in this category expend more energy on maladaptive activities and have only limited energy available for combatting stress or engaging in productive activity.

The labile personality has a greater chance of developing hypertension. Such a person is subject to *labile hypertension* – when he is heavily stressed his blood pressure rises into the hypertensive range, but when that stress is removed it returns to normal. This situation occurs because the mind is not harmonized with and, therefore, is not strong enough to control the pranas and the autonomic nervous system, so that they go out of balance in any stressful situation.

Gellhorn and Kiely have shown that lability of the autonomic nervous system leads to hypertension via increased sympathetic tone.[4] David Orme-Johnson, a psychologist at the University of Texas, USA, has demonstrated improved autonomic stability, decreased anxiety (and therefore better resistance to stress) in those people who practised meditation.[5] Wallace and Benson have also pointed out that meditators have a more stable personality and are less prone to disease.

The endocrines and personality

Before we attempt to explain how the endocrine glands affect hypertension there are a few basic points which must be understood. Endocrine glands are those which secrete chemicals, called hormones, directly into the bloodstream. This is opposed to the exocrine glands which secrete chemicals via ducts onto surfaces such as the skin, bowel walls and so on. Hormones have specific effects on the metabolism and activity of certain body organs. There are seven major endocrine glands: the pituitary, pineal, thyroid and parathyroid, thymus, pancreas, adrenals and gonads (sex glands). The status of the thymus as an endocrine gland is controversial, but it is included for completeness.

Endocrines are one of the more interesting fields of medicine because of their direct link with personality and

46

character and their connection with the psychic centres (chakras) at the higher levels of our being.

For the personality to be balanced and healthy, the endocrine glands must be balanced within themselves and with the rest of the body. Most of these glands are believed to be controlled by a master gland, the pituitary, though research in this field is showing that the pineal gland may even control the pituitary. The pituitary and the pineal have direct links to the brain so there is an endocrine-nervous system interaction for better control and integration of the body. When the endocrine glands are not balanced, disease can result because both body and personality are affected adversely. In hypertensive disease we are especially concerned with imbalance of the adrenal and thyroid glands and, in turn, their imbalance with the nervous system.

At the physical level the endocrine glands monitor the internal body secretions and ensure that just the right level of hormone is in the blood. One molecule of adrenaline can affect the whole body. It has been estimated that if we were to tip one ounce of adrenaline into a small lake and ensure that it were mixed properly and then inject some lake water into a person, we would get the response typical of adrenaline secretion from the adrenal glands. It only takes minute quantities to have an enormous effect on the physical and more subtle bodies. Any imbalance in the endocrine glands can cause excess secretions, especially when the body is responding to stresses, and has vast repercussions.

It has been known for some time that the brain is protected from certain chemicals in the blood by a blood/brain barrier. This is a semi-permeable membrane which permits only special molecules, such as oxygen and glucose (food), to pass through. The pituitary, so-called 'master gland,' was thought to be protected by this barrier. Recently it has been found that this barrier is broken at the pituitary. A small part at the front of the gland is exposed directly to the bloodstream. Any food or substance we put into the blood will affect the pituitary and thus the whole endocrinal system. This means

47

that the treatment of disease will have to be re-evaluated to ensure the drugs used do not affect the endocrine balance.

At a more subtle level, the seven major chakras correspond to the endocrine system of the physical body. The classical picture is: pituitary – sahasrara; pineal – ajna; thyroid – vishuddhi; thymus – anahata; adrenals – manipura, gonads – swadhisthana; perineal body – mooladhara.

These points are also the locations of nerve plexes which create a nerve-hormone-chakra complex, and at these points energy flows into the body. You can imagine such a point as being formed by a needle and thread sewing the mental, pranic and physical bodies together. It is the intersection of mind and body energies. Mental energy directs pranic energy in the physical body. In disease, a disordered mind and a cluttered, complex personality cannot direct energy effectively in a balanced, harmonious way. One can see the repercussions on the endocrine level when we consider that a person with excessive hormone secretion from the thyroid gland is anxious and irritable, and shows all the signs of mental imbalance in the hyperactive direction. The reverse situation of low thyroid function gives lethargy, depression, apathy and a general slowing of mental abilities.

Any imbalance of mind reflects into the endocrines and vice versa. This imbalance creates disease but is not a disease entity in itself. It is one of the causative factors. Many people have a slight hormonal imbalance in the neuro-endocrine axis. This is evidenced at the social level by preoccupation with sexuality (linked to the gonad-swadhisthana interaction) and power-seeking, competition and lack of regard for others (caused by imbalances in the adrenal-manipura interaction). This imbalance affects the pituitary and thus all the endocrine glands of the body are affected.

Endocrine glands and hypertension
Hypertension is the outcome of long-term nervous hormonal and pranic imbalance which in turn causes the adrenal glands to secrete excess adrenaline and noradrenaline.

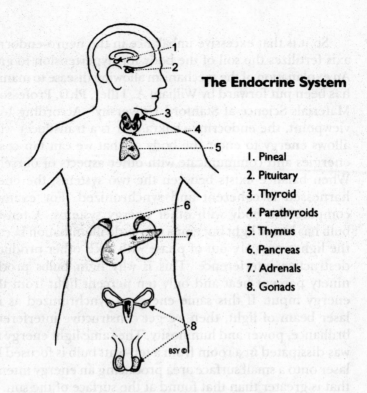

The Endocrine System

1. Pineal
2. Pituitary
3. Thyroid
4. Parathyroids
5. Thymus
6. Pancreas
7. Adrenals
8. Gonads

BSY ©

Adrenaline causes increased respiration, heart rate and blood pressure; blood is shifted to the brain, heart and muscles from the digestive system; sugar is released from the liver; the spleen contracts, releasing blood cells; hairs stand on end; and the pupils of the eyes dilate to let in as much light as possible. The body is prepared to face stress or to run away from it; this is the 'fight or flight' mechanism. *Noradrenaline* seems only to increase the blood pressure.

Daniel Funkenstein examined the role of these two hormones in hypertension[6] and found that excess adrenaline was secreted in those people with high blood pressure whose personality expressed their inner anger through depression. Noradrenaline was predominant in those who expressed anger openly. Also, aggressive animals, such as lions or tigers, have higher levels of noradrenaline. Passive ones such as the rabbit have higher levels of adrenaline.

49

So it is that excessive imbalance in the neuro-endocrine axis fertilizes the soil of the body for hypertension to grow. An explanation of the mechanism allowing disease to manifest has been put forward by William A. Tiller, PhD, Professor of Materials Science at Stanford University[7]. According to his viewpoint, the endocrine-chakra pair is a transducer which allows energy to enter the body so that we can tap cosmic energies and communicate with other aspects of ourselves. When balance exists between the two systems, the energy harnessed is coherent and synchronized. For example, compare the body with other energy systems. A ten-watt bulb has lots of light but emits very little illumination because the light waves are out of phase with each other producing destructive interference. This is why light bulbs produce ninety percent heat and only ten percent light from their energy input. If this same energy is synchronized as in a laser beam of light, then we get constructive interference, brilliance, power and luminosity. The same light energy that was dissipated in a room from a ten-watt bulb is focused by a laser onto a small surface area producing an energy intensity that is greater than that found at the surface of the sun.

Destructive interference describes the situation in the hypertensive person and constructive interference applies to the ideal. In the real situation most people are somewhere between the two extremes and tend more towards the destructive side when they become ill. The constructive interference picture describes the yogi who – having mastered the body, emotions and mind – can concentrate the energies in his chakras to the point where the energy available approaches the infinite resources of the cosmos. Without this yogic control people tend to function at low energy levels. Their chakras, which are psychic energy vortices, spin erratically and unevenly, so that some are switched on, while others are switched off. This occurs because the energy flowing into them has to move through impure channels which are sometimes blocked either partially or wholly. This is analogous to a hose plugged into a rotating sprinkler

Chakra-Endocrine Complex

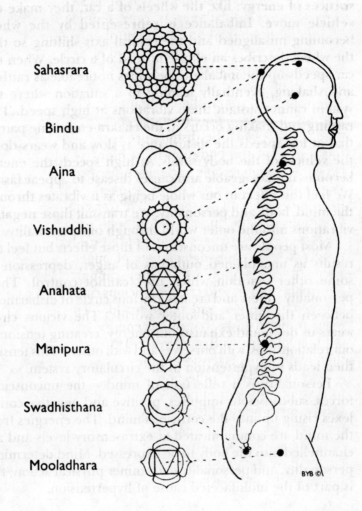

Sahasrara

Bindu

Ajna

Vishuddhi

Anahata

Manipura

Swadhisthana

Mooladhara

BYB ©

system. If the hose or sprinkler is blocked the rotation is impeded, preventing distribution of water to nourish the earth. When the erratic pattern continues in the body for a long period, disease can result. Impurities build up in the physical and pranic body, due to damming up of energy in the chakras and the channels feeding them.

51

The word *chakra* means 'wheel'. Chakras are spinning vortices of energy; like the wheels of a car, they make the vehicle move. Imbalance is represented by the wheel becoming misaligned and the central axis shifting so that the wheel describes an ellipse instead of a circle. When the car speeds up the imbalance becomes noticeable as rattling and shaking, eventually leading to a situation where the system cannot sustain these vibrations at high speed. This rattling and shaking occurs in the chakra-endocrine pair so that at low speeds the disturbance is slow and wears down the vehicle of the body slowly. At high speeds the energy becomes unmanageable and causes disease to appear faster. We feel this effect in our whole being as it vibrates through the mind, body and personality. We transmit those negative vibrations into the outer world through our personality.

Most people are unconscious of those effects but feel the results as unexplained outbursts of anger, depression or some other emotion which they cannot control. Their personality suffers and creates a vicious circle of disharmony between the inner and outer worlds. The vicious circle wears us down and exhausts our energy, creating tension in our relationships, with ourselves and with others. This tension then leads to hypertension in the circulatory system.

Personality is a reflection of mind – the unconscious forces, subconscious impulses, positive and negative complexes rising up into the conscious mind. The energies from the mind are communicated at extrasensory levels and are channelled into the body to be expressed. Mind determines personality, and personality determines physical action; this is part of the multifaceted cause of hypertension.

Lifestyle

The mind is the basis of our way of living in the world. From the mind come thoughts, from thoughts come actions. Those lead to daily habits which pattern our existence, and establish the framework around which we work and act throughout the day and night. The habits, desires and ambitions of life modify the essential qualities of life, creating for each of us our own little universe. It is this universe which determines what we achieve in life and whether we are healthy or unhealthy.

Swami Sivananda of Rishikesh has summed up this process perfectly in the following poem:

> Sow a thought and reap an action.
> Sow an action and reap a habit.
> Sow a habit and reap a character.
> Sow a character and reap a destiny.

Today's lifestyle is not based on scientific principles and this is reflected in the increased amount of spectator sports, such as television-watching, cinema and newspapers. Today's lifestyle is not in harmony with the world around us, and therefore the destiny we reap causes suffering.

Diet and sleep are not scheduled to harmonize with the light and dark cycles of the day, seasons, temperature, climate and so on. People eat too much and sleep too long. The average modern diet and sleep patterns are unhealthy in quality and quantity. Too much sleep leaves us still feeling tired and unable to get out of bed in the morning, while too much food makes us feel heavy and full, increasing the grosser aspects of our existence. All these predispose us to ill health and high blood pressure over a period of time.

One example of this disharmony occurs when you are tense and lead a fast lifestyle. You do not have time to breathe correctly. The cycle of breathing is not harmonized with the rest of the body or with environmental cycles. Thus we may take enough oxygen in, but breathe too quickly to allow efficient transfer of oxygen in the blood to take place. Or we may not breathe deeply enough and therefore not bring enough oxygen into the lungs. Shallow inefficient respiration reflects mental tension and leads to chronic fatigue and low prana shakti.

When the process of breathing incorrectly becomes chronic, we set the scene for physical and mental tensions to spiral into chronically raised blood pressure. This pathologically elevated blood pressure is a reflection of our lifestyle where we are not aware of our own bodies, breath or minds, nor of the consequences of this ignorance. Incorrect breathing becomes a habit with us, a habit that must be broken through the practice of pranayama.

Another example of the imbalance of cycles and internal rhythms is that of passengers on east-west air flights who experience 'time-lag' and an unpleasant readjustment phase.

Van Bount, Gangon, et al. have found that light enters our brains through some other means than the eyes and affects hormone cycles.[8] It is believed that light may influence the menstrual cycle. Man responds to solar and lunar cycles, but he is rarely aware of those rhythms. Living in the city a person may not see the moon for months on end, and may remain unaware of its constant but subtle forces which are difficult to perceive in the jostle of our daily lives.

Much human behaviour is the result of conditioned behaviour patterns implanted in the brain and mind, especially during childhood. These may persist unmodified, but more often become gradually adapted to changes and influences in the environment.

Habits force us to react in predetermined and fixed fashions to life's situations. If we desire something and are able to satisfy the desire we are happy for a while, but if the desire is not fulfilled we are dissatisfied, and frustration arises. This frustration creates inner tension. For example, if we are late for work or caught in a traffic jam, we become tense because we are anxious to be elsewhere and do not like to be stuck in the middle of town. We cannot relax. We have learned the habit of anxious reaction, but we have not learned the habit of relaxation.

The result of inner tension is to turn on sympathetic nervous system activity. Because so much of our lives is frustrated by a fast-moving, polluted and stress-laden society, inner tension rises.

K.S. Gopal, researcher into the yogic management of hypertension, states:

"There have been tremendous changes in the environment and conditions of living of human beings. There is good reason to believe that in those changing environments, incessant stimulation of the sympathetic nervous system is largely responsible for the high incidence of hypertension and other similar serious diseases."[9]

A stressful lifestyle affects every aspect of our existence. As we can see from the following statistics:

- One third of American males have hypertension.
- One half of deaths in America are from heart and circulatory diseases.
- In 1970 five billion doses of tranquilizers, five billion doses of barbiturates and three billion doses of amphetamines were manufactured.
- In the same year, doctors wrote over 200 million prescriptions for the above drugs, all of which are habit-forming and to be used only when absolutely necessary.

The above situation is frightening in terms of its huge proportion and it is typical of most western technologically advancing countries. It is more frightening when you think that the stress which requires such an enormous supply of tranquilizing drugs is not being eliminated by modern science but actually increasing.

Drugs not only fail to cure high blood pressure and remove the stress that causes it but, in fact, compound the problem by interfering with natural body rhythms. They also disturb sleep patterns, shutting off the dreaming phase responsible for releasing stresses. Drugs only remove the overt symptoms. To remove the cause at its roots requires meditation. This is because meditation deals directly with the mind in which lie the roots of all psychosomatic diseases, as well as hypertension.

If you suffer from hypertension or any disease or discomfort then you are suffering from negative programming. This program has been built into our neuronal brain circuits throughout our lives. Of course there are positive circuits too, but the negative and painful circuits, those that cause mental and emotional suffering, seem to stand out more in our minds than the positive. Yet this situation can be rectified through yogic practices of awareness and deconditioning.

It is lack of awareness in our lifestyle which has created the conditions for cultivation of hypertension. Many people are unconscious of the stored tensions within although everyone has them. This means that the lack of awareness extends deep into the five koshas (body sheaths): body, emotions, mind, psyche and spirit. We are not aware of ourselves and ignorance results in habits detrimental to our health. If we really knew the harm we are doing to ourselves with these habits we would immediately eliminate them. The wisdom and power to do this arise from the knowledge and understanding we gain through yoga.

Heredity and Ageing

It is medically proven that people who have a family history of high blood pressure are more likely to suffer from this disease. The two components of this observation are heredity and environment. Environment refers to the atmosphere is which our parents and others have reared us, plus our later lifestyle and interpersonal relationships. Those modify the inherent and basic characteristics passed on to us by our parents through genetic heredity. The way we live and how we modify our lives so as to reinforce or improve weak points in our bodies will determine how we age, whether our arteries harden quickly, slowly or not at all and whether our blood pressure rises to abnormal levels or remains at healthy levels.

Heredity

Genes make up chromosomes which are the blueprint for the basic body structure and its constitution. The combination of genes from our parents determines individual characteristics such as height, hair colour and so on. Weaknesses can also be inherited and it is at these weakest points in the body that disease will manifest; it is the weak link in the chain that will break. Heredity predetermines where this weak point is going to be, but it does not mean that we will necessarily break at this point. Genetic structure only lays down some of the channels of least resistance, allowing the body energies to flow in certain directions.

Whether or not illness eventuates in weak areas depends very much on whether we live in a healthy or unhealthy environment from birth onwards.

The environment modifies our hereditary tendencies. If we live in a supportive environment, one that tends to make us healthy and gives mental strength and balance, then we will be able to correct the deficiencies in our body and overcome the obstacles on the path to good health. On the other hand, if we live in a negative environment, we tend to be caught in negative cycles. Those wear us down both physically and mentally, and accentuate any inherited tendency towards high blood pressure.

The brain is linked directly to the mind. Energy flows into the brain and is channelled through billions of neuronal circuits, which are primarily determined by heredity. Environmental and inner experiences modify these circuits and create fine enveloping and organizing webs for the mind and inherited patterns to work through. The more frequently a pathway in the brain is used, the stronger nerve connections become. If the circuit is not used it tends to be dominated by other circuits whose actions are reinforced.

The fact that the neuronal circuits of the brain are ever changing and subject to the environment and lifestyle has been proved in experiments. When animals, raised from birth in environments where they could see only vertical bars, were placed in a normal environment, they could only avoid the vertical bars. They could not see, and therefore could not avoid, horizontal bars. Later, their brains grew to suit the environment as new areas in the visual cortex began to open up.

The structure of the nerve pathways is built up by experience and can be changed according to new experiences. The brain actually develops most of its circuits in the first few years of life, for the major areas of the nervous system are not formed at birth and must be learned. Only certain instinctual reflexes are present at birth. It seems, then, that heredity plays a minor role in hypertension because experience and the things we learn from our parents are the more important factors in our behaviour. If your parents are hypertensive then you grow in this atmosphere and develop the same patterns of thought and behaviour.

The hereditary patterns of the brain are such that certain individuals tend to channel energy into the blood vessel system so that hypertension results. If this tendency is reinforced by the environment and lifestyle then disease manifests in the course of time.

Ageing

With increasing age there is an increased chance of the arteries hardening and the blood pressure rising irreversibly. This only occurs if the lifestyle and lack of self-discipline create the conditions. If you have looked after your body and kept your mind strong, young and alert, there is every chance that you will not develop hypertension and will live a healthy, relaxed and peaceful existence.

Mind, prana, lifestyle and heredity determine how fast we age. If our mind is relaxed and stable, capable of responding to the world and handling the pressures of life, then we age gracefully and maintain a young and healthy appearance. We have all seen people who are sixty years of age and look thirty. If we are mentally tense, then our bodies tense, the muscles tighten and the blood vessels and all tissues are adversely affected. Tissues deteriorate and age faster. We have also seen people who are thirty years of age and look sixty. In this situation pranic energy cannot work well as it does not have a good machine to work with. The pranic energy flow slows down, the chakras spin slower and more erratically, channels become blocked or dislocated and function deteriorates. Hereditary factors accentuate the process of mental stress and thereby direct the destructive energy to cause hypertension, which is found to be most common in the elderly.

In modern society there is the tendency for blood pressure to increase with age, though the reason is not known. The reason is probably tied up with the effect of ageing on the tissues so that blood vessels become harder and less flexible, and so the pressure inside them tends to rise. The process implies degeneration. This is the opposite of the situation that occurs in yoga, where the tissues age but do not deteriorate. Instead they become stronger with age. Too often, however, our bodies decay even before we die. The modern urban lifestyle accelerates the ageing process and the tendency to develop degenerative diseases such as high blood pressure.

The Total View

A neurosis has really come to an end when it has overcome the wrongly oriented ego. The neurosis itself is not healed; it heals us. The man is ill, but the illness is an attempt of nature to heal him. We can therefore learn a great deal for the good of our health from the illness itself, and that which appears to the neurotic person as absolutely to be rejected is just the part which contains the true gold which we should otherwise never have found.

C.G. Jung

We have divided the cause of hypertension into various modes and compartments. These describe the route by which energies from the mind enter the body and from there travel out again into the world and universe around us, to be reflected back onto us once more in a cyclical fashion. There is no true separation. The process is a unified one. The mind, emotions, body, world and universe are one organism when seen from the expanded point of view obtained through yoga. Hypertension is the result of many factors but these factors spring from one undeniable fact at the base of our existence. That fact is ignorance *(avidya)*.

Ignorance is the cause of all disease and knowledge is the cure. When we get sick it is a signal from nature that something is not right. It is a warning to change ourselves. Because of our ignorance we have not been aware of the processes going on within us that have led to hypertension.

61

We have a distorted view of the way we are and how we should live. We do not know who we are. To learn we have to suffer and go through the pain of life. What yoga allows us to do is to remove the hurt from the pain so that we can grow with each experience whether 'good' or 'bad.'

We are living, growing organisms in an infinite universe. To grow truly and become really human we must go through the life process. Some suffer mentally, emotionally or spiritually; some get hypertension and others get ulcers. This is all a part of our schooling here on earth. Paradoxically, some of us must get sick to learn about ourselves more fully and completely.

When we look at hypertension from this perspective it is clear that there is a cure. When we have studied the situation we will know and understand how it came about. Then we can alter our lives and ourselves. When we have learned our lesson, the hypertension will disappear. The true cause of hypertension is ignorance of the mind, the physical body and the whole human vehicle; ignorance of why we are on this planet and how to live the right way.

As all great philosophies have said throughout time and space: "Know thyself" and "Unto thine own self be true". This is the essence of yoga and it is how yoga has come to understand the cause of, and the cure for, hypertension.

Cure

Yogic Cure

This is dedicated to those who suffer from stress. To those who in their efforts for good or evil, for peace or war, have sustained wounds, loss of blood or exposure to extremes of temperature, hunger, fatigue, want of air, infections, poisons or deadly rays. To those who are under the exhausting nervous strain of pursuing their ideal – whatever it may be. To the martyrs who sacrifice themselves for others, as well as to those hounded by selfish ambition, fear, jealousy and worst of all, hate. For my stress stems from the urge to help and not to judge. I understand that I cannot and should not be cured of my stress but merely taught to understand it.

Dr Hans Selye

Yoga aims to remove hypertension and its potentially lethal effects through a system of asanas (poses), pranayama (breathing exercises) and meditation, along with a complete reappraisal of lifestyle. Through this you gain a new dimension of meaning in your life and begin to see the world around you with new eyes, revaluing and restructuring your existence, bringing order out of chaos. In this way you remove mental disease that often leads to physical disease.

Yoga helps you to build up physical resistance, emotional harmony and pranic balance through the eradication of the root cause in the mind. Asanas and pranayama help in this process of self-healing. In this way you also gain the satisfaction of knowing that you can achieve what may have once appeared to be impossible – the cure of hypertension.

The neo-industrial age is also called the age of anxiety. Life is full of subtle psychological plagues, worries, vague conflicts, loneliness, disillusionment and doubt. Stress and psychological disease are now firmly part of our lifestyle, and affluent nations are especially prone to suffer from the effects of acute stress. The main reason for this is the unawareness of the spiritual reality within that gives a deeper meaning to life.

It is only when we find meaning in life that we can cure hypertension fully in all its subtle forms. When meaning enters our life we relax because we begin to find satisfaction and fulfilment. Everything, no matter how small, takes on importance and has its own special place in our lives. This reflects in our mental and physical circuits and creates order from chaos, toning down the sympathetic nervous system and adrenal oversecretion, thereby removing the excessive peripheral resistance in our blood vessels and the effects of stress from our bodies.

Yoga helps you to cure yourself from hypertension by offering the following practices:

1. *Relaxation techniques* which incorporate desensitization, autosuggestion, and deconditioning to remove mental tensions and complexes. These practices help you to cultivate a positive attitude towards life and yourself. Each experience then becomes a learning process even if there is a little pain involved. Through awareness you replace mistaken concepts with more realistic, practical and positive concepts of life.

2. *Asana and pranayama* rebalance the physical, emotional, pranic, mental and psychic aspects of being.

3. *Meditation* induces relaxation and develops self-knowledge. Your awareness moves inward, away from external stress and influences, cleaning out the mind step by step, purifying, remoulding and realizing more and more about yourself. Meditation follows from sense withdrawal

66

(*pratyahara*) and concentration (*dharana*), and finally culminates in self-realization.

The awareness is dissociated from the physical body and made one-pointed, inducing a meditative state in which alpha and theta waves are produced by the brain. They indicate deep relaxation and spontaneous creativity. The activity of the brain slows down allowing a state of complete rest to occur in the body and mind. The breath and heart rate are lowered, and the whole body enjoys deep rest. In this state the blood vessels dilate and oxygenated pure blood reaches the body organs, rejuvenating and repairing damaged tissues and maintaining healthy tissue. Lactate and other toxic poisons are removed more efficiently and the vitality increases. The circuits of the brain and mind are given the chance to reshape themselves into a more harmonious form which affects the whole body through the peripheral nervous system.

4. *Kundalini kriyas* are a powerful means of activating prana shakti in the body so that the pranic channels, the nadis, are charged and cleaned of impurities which impede the flow of energy. They rebalance the sympathetic and parasympathetic nervous systems, and reintegrate the endocrine glands. This brings the adrenal glands back into their proper place so they do not secrete excessive amounts of hormones which increase blood pressure. Control over these mechanisms becomes more precise.

It has been found that all of the above yogic practices aid in the cure of hypertension by:

• Reducing mental tension.
• Rebalancing and enriching your supply of prana.
• Removing the effects of stress, such as toxic wastes.
• Reharmonizing the endocrine-chakra complex.
• Adjusting your lifestyle so that it becomes more positive and healthy, removing the bad habits that have led to high blood pressure, such as smoking, overeating, oversleeping, fast-living and insufficient exercise.

- Strengthening the whole mind-body complex so that hereditary and acquired weaknesses are removed. The ageing process slows and does not result in tissue degeneration. Rather, tissues are regenerated through meditation, redirection of prana and healthy life habits.

Yogic lifestyle

These practices are eventually incorporated into a yogic lifestyle, a lifestyle based on the scientific understanding and practical experience of yogis through the ages. When this is achieved, the effects accumulate and add up to decreased blood pressure. If you continue to maintain the old habits that are detrimental to your health then you lessen the positive benefits that accrue from regular practice of yogic techniques. Most people find, however, that they feel good after doing yogic sadhana (practices) and naturally and gradually readjust their lives so that they maintain their positive frame of mind and bodily health. In this way they overcome the effects of heredity and environment and transmute the 'growing old' process into a 'growing' and learning experience.

Awareness of limitations

An old warrior had just returned from a battle carrying with him the spoils of his endeavour. Because of the weight of the loot he decided to sell some of his exquisite treasures.

"Will you buy this trusty sword?" he asked a traveller. "Only ten pieces of gold." The traveller immediately snapped up the bargain.

The warrior's companion could not believe his eyes. As soon as the transaction was completed he asked, "Why did you only ask ten pieces of gold for that priceless sword?"

The old warrior replied, "I have only ten fingers. Is there any number higher than ten?"

We are limited by our thoughts and beliefs. These same limitations applied to running the four minute mile until it was broken. The same applies to the hypertensive situation today. The medical profession knows no cure for it yet, so most people believe that there is no cure for hypertension, just as the seller of the sword could not imagine a number greater than ten because no one had told him that higher numbers existed. This situation creates a fixed mental attitude which makes it more difficult for people to cure themselves.

To cure hypertension we must first know the correct method in order to achieve positive results. Firstly, we have to realize that cure is possible and then we have to proceed along the yogic path which leads to that cure. Through yoga you will come to realize that many of the thoughts and beliefs we hold are founded on ignorance and fear. We build up customs and habits and find it very difficult to change them even when a better and healthier system comes along. It is only when the social beliefs and cultural habits no longer serve the needs of the people and have done their damage that there is a public outcry and a frantic search for alternatives. Today this need is apparent when we look at the situation of hypertension, a malady which is wasting so much manpower and valuable potential in our society. Yoga offers practical explanations as to what is wrong with the present lifestyle and how we can solve these problems.

The fact that there is a problem in world health was pointed out by Prof L.K. White in a survey of the USA, Canada, the UK, Switzerland, Yugoslavia, Finland, Poland and Argentina. He questioned about 48,000 people representing 15,000,000 people, and the survey did not include patients in hospital or other health institutions.[10] White classified people into three categories:

1. *Unhealthy:*
   a) inability to carry out social duties
   b) detectable known illness
   c) physiological symptoms of illness, such as cough, chest pain, shortness of breath, stiffness, anxiety and swelling of joints
   d) dental morbidity
   e) perceptual visual defects.

69

2. *Functionally healthy*: Though able to work and not confined to bed, these people reported some slight or chronic,
but not disabling, ailment and manifested one or more of
the above signs to a slight degree.
3. *Healthy*: These people had none of the above signs. The
results showed that only 14.3 percent were healthy, 24.4
percent were functionally healthy and 61.3 percent were
unhealthy. Thus an astronomical number of people in
the world today suffer illness of some kind, are chronically
disabled, physically impaired, handicapped, or have long-
standing bad health resulting in some disability. Of those
with poor health, one of the largest groups is sufferers of
hypertension.

This problem of worldwide bad health has arisen because
people have not been taught to take responsibility for their
actions. We act without spontaneity, abiding by self-imposed
limitations and fears. We live our life and suffer the
consequences, whether we are prepared to do so or not. We
must learn to overcome negative forces so that they do not
manipulate and manoeuvre our lives.

Yoga gives us the methods and techniques to build up
the willpower and mental strength to combat the habits that
produce tension and disease. This is the direct way to self-
mastery and harmonious, healthy living.

Eliminating Mental Problems

By removing mental problems we remove the causative factors that have led to hypertension. This is achieved by freeing the mind of chaos and turmoil so that it can think more clearly and function more efficiently. Problems that seem insoluble in a state of tension are easily solved when the mind is relaxed. The following points can help in the process of relaxation and should be combined with traditional yogic practices:

- When a child sleeps he forgets all his problems and really sleeps. When he plays, full attention is given to the present moment, free from worries and cares of past and future. Try to cultivate this present-centred awareness. Most worries and anxieties are imaginary and exaggerated from the reality. By relaxing you can better cope with any problem, and also develop self-confidence.

- Your mind has a great reserve of power within the subconscious and unconsciousness. It can solve many problems for you without the need for thought at a conscious level, but only if you relax and let the deeper process function. Feed the data into your mind as you would a computer, and the answer will appear intuitively at the right time and place. This process is enhanced by faith and trust in the workings of our deeper self.

- When something disturbs your mind, do not get involved in it. Be a witness, an observer and just watch the process

71

going on. All thoughts carry energy or prana; becoming involved with them creates emotions and waves in the mind. Cultivate your witness consciousness and you can extricate yourself from the mire you have been involved in up to now. This cuts down the wear and tear that negative emotional energy has on the body in terms of sympathetic overstimulation and its resultant increase in blood pressure.

- Accept yourself and your feelings. Do not compare yourself with any other person. Remember that each person has his own talent and outstanding features. By doing what is natural for you, you will achieve the best results you can and fit more harmoniously into the whole. This will have a soothing effect on your mind and bring the blood pressure down. Do not be deceived by appearances. Most people put up a front for others, yet within they too have the same problems, faults and feelings as you.

- Look within for happiness. People in a materialistic culture usually seek happiness outside of themselves rather than inside. When we look within, we find the true source of happiness.

- Learn to accept your inner feelings and emotions without any feeling of guilt. Act out these inner responses to external situations, but be aware at each moment of why and what you are doing. Anger, greed, jealousy and other negative mental forces are a part of most people's makeup and experience. When we examine carefully what is going on inside, this is what we see. Tantric philosophy suggests that one should suppress nothing and accept everything, both good and bad. You can rise by skilfully using what makes you fall and suffer. Instincts are a part of human nature, so we must accept them. In this way we slowly come to understand our inner self and evolve into a higher sphere of understanding. Come to know yourself and enjoy your own company, as if you were your own best friend.

72

- Cultivate yourself. When you have accepted what you are and come to know those things that have been hidden within you for so long, correct your faults and master your lower nature. This is achieved slowly, step by step and if possible with guidance. You are a tree and must be nourished by cultivating those things which make you healthy.
- Do not feel guilty about the past. Shakespeare said, "What's gone and what's past should be past grief". The past is finished, so learn from your mistakes and in future know that you will not repeat them. In this way you can improve your present. If you keep your past in the present, you only clutter up your mind and make yourself unhappy. Enjoy every moment of the day.
- Try to be open to people, even if you do not like what you see. Each person has something to teach us, and you can learn a lot from difficult situations. Remember that other people have their problems too, and perhaps it is possible for you to help that person overcome a problem and so progress to a more mature personality. Everyone has the potential to help us to reach higher consciousness if we are receptive.
- Discover your greatest needs, attachments, desires, and try to reduce your need to find happiness in the outside environment. Look within yourself. In this way you will foster self-reliance, independence of both thought and action, and flexibility.

These attitudes are fostered by and enhance yoga practices to combat mental problems. The practices themselves effect a most powerful change in the mind, and those most appropriate to hypertension are desensitization, auto-suggestion, deconditioning and detachment. These practices are ideally used when you are completely relaxed, for instance, after yoga practice, in yoga nidra, or just before and after sleep. When the mind is relaxed it is more receptive and can change faster and more easily.

73

Desensitization

You have a problem and you can see it clearly but are unable to remove it. The solution to the problem eludes you. What can you do? Many people become involved in complex and usually unsuitable methods in an attempt to avoid the problem altogether. Yet, with the application of yogic common sense, the answer is easier than you might think.

Become aware that you have this problem, the implications of it in your life, and its effects. Then tell yourself mentally, "I do not care if I have a problem or not." That is, do not let it affect you. It can stay or go as it likes, but you are determined not to be involved or affected by it. This will remove the negative effect it has on your mind and allow you to learn from the experience.

When these effects are removed, the energy tied up in the problem is discharged. As you relax during your practice, bring that problem directly into your consciousness. Confront it, whether it be a fear, an obsession or whatever. Visualize the object or situation, and fully experience the feeling of fear, anger, anxiety as the case may be.

At first the intensity of the experience will be great, for new channels must open up to release the energy behind our feelings. Yet, just as a carbonated drink fizzes when it is first opened and then slowly subsides, so with continued daily practice the emotional response is lessened.

Ensure that when you practise, you are quite relaxed. Watch the effects on your body and mind. This technique is especially recommended for the more obvious and conscious disturbances. In this way you will remove many of the problems that are causing the excessive sympathetic stimulation and adrenal oversecretion which produce high blood pressure.

Autosuggestion

This technique can be used together with desensitization. Autosuggestion is a very powerful technique and most people use it every day without realizing it. You will hear the

74

following words: 'He makes me sick,' 'I nearly died' or 'I knew that would go wrong.' This sort of thinking, though apparently harmless, is negative and these seemingly innocuous suggestions deeply affect the subconscious mind. Every action, thought and word is registered by the powerful, hidden aspects of the mind and their action on our lives is not consciously felt until we try to cultivate awareness through the practices of yoga.

Autosuggestion can also be used to bring awareness of the workings of the mind. Once you have experienced the way this technique works for yourself, you will fully understand the limitless potential that exists in each of us and what can be achieved by those who learn to develop their awareness.

Whether you make your suggestion without any awareness, as most people do, or with awareness – it does not matter. The process will still continue and its effects will be felt. In the first case you will not understand what is happening, but when you make the suggestion with a purpose in your mind you can easily determine what effects are related to what cause. To become responsible for your actions you must realize how it is that you create your life through your own thoughts. Make your thoughts work for you by using autosuggestion.

By making a *sankalpa*, a resolve, we use autosuggestion to reprogram the mind so that, over some time, the whole being is changed in a positive way. This technique is best used in such states as yoga nidra, which is like the feeling you have just before you go to sleep. A sankalpa is a short, positive statement of your own choice that is charged with feeling and determination and planted deep within the subconscious mind. The statement may be 'I will become more aware,' ' will work for the good of humanity' or 'I will overcome all obstacles'. Visualize the positive mental attitude you wish to develop. For example, in a fear-provoking situation, see yourself acting with courage based on mature understanding of the true situation.

75

Deconditioning

Mental problems exist because of conditioning, a train of suggestions which has been going on since birth. Even while you were in the womb you were subject to conditioning from your mother's internal reactions to her environment. You are at the mercy of the way your mind has been repeatedly conditioned to act in certain situations. This conditioning is recorded in the neuronal circuits of the brain as well as within the personality. At one moment you may be calm and at the next moment emotionally upset, angry or depressed because some trivial factor has triggered mental and neuronal brain circuits so that you act in a conditioned way. These circuits were formed by your heredity and the environment. You have learned these responses from parents, friends and society, and because of *samskaras* (impressions) in the depths of your personality.

The brain is a fantastic tool. It has some fifteen billion cells. Each cell has an estimated 500,000 connections. Though the brain weighs only two percent of the total body weight, it receives seventeen percent of the body's supply of blood and consumes ten percent of the body's oxygen. It is beyond the comprehension of man's present day intellect to fathom its workings. To profit by and fully utilize this computer we have to learn the basic mechanisms underlying its structure. Through yoga practices we can develop this awareness. Until now we have allowed our brain to be polluted with much useless and unnecessary information which distorts the purity of its function. Remove the impurities and unnecessary programs from your mind and you will remove them from the brain's circuits.

Remove the programs of fear, insecurity, anger, alienation and feelings of helplessness. Become aware of your thoughts, ideas and beliefs and realize that they are a part of your past conditioning. Gain this through meditation, contemplation, remembrance of past events and awareness. We are only aware of a small fraction of the millions of bits of information coming into our brains every second of the day. The eye has

76

two million nerve connections and the ears have several hundred thousand, but we are aware of only a small fraction of the information they carry. We are only aware of a fragment of every moment, and lost moments are gone forever.

Try to be aware of those things that happened to you in the past that you have forgotten but which still exert an influence over you at the subconscious level. An example of negative programming is that of the child who wanders near a busy road. The mother sees this, becomes emotional and scolds the child. The child is only aware that the person he feels closest to and is totally dependent on is distraught and hitting him, sending out bad vibrations. The mother is acting in accordance with her conditioning which has resulted in fear and anxiety and is programming her child in the same way. The effects on the child are negative and will continue to have an influence as he grows up. He will therefore respond to stressful situations in the same way, with fear, shouting, anger and other negative emotions, all of which can have a detrimental effect on his health and produce high blood pressure.

In this connection, there is the story of a Zen master who one day asked his pupil a question. When the disciple answered the master was pleased. The next day the master asked the same question and received the same reply. This time he became very angry. Why? Because his disciple had answered automatically, in a conditioned, unthinking way.

Yoga removes this conditioning by extending awareness over our whole lives so that we gain insight into our motives, thoughts, beliefs and actions. As you become more aware you will feel carefree, peaceful and clear in thought, perception and decision. You will experience a tremendous agility and flexibility in every facet of life, from the very movement of the physical body to the freedom in your ability to communicate with and respond appropriately to people. In this way you will snuff out the illusory dream world of the past that has coloured your perception of the world around you and led to hypertension.

77

Detachment

When you decondition the mind you empty it of complexes, neuroses and so on. Do not recondition it and thereby defeat the purpose. The mind should remain like a mirror, reflecting each situation clearly and giving the true response without the fog of ego, conditioning and so on.

There is another story of a man who visits a Zen master in search of satori, enlightenment. The master offers him tea and starts to fill the cup, but when the cup is full he continues pouring so that the tea spills everywhere. The visitor cries out, "Stop, stop!" The master says, "How can I pour new knowledge and understanding into a head that is already full of so much rubbish?"

Try to be an observer under all circumstances, even the most tumultuous, frenzied, agitated or disturbing circumstances. You will learn that you are not what you do; that is, you are not a doctor, a plumber, an engineer, a housewife. You are something quite different from that. Without this awareness you tend to become trapped within your role in life, and all the ups and downs. Your body and mind are constantly changing, so you are not these either. Try to find what is permanent and immortal within you through the practice of detachment with relaxation and awareness.

Practise detachment and you will be like a rubber ball, resilient and strong enough to bounce through every difficult situation in life, rather than being a delicate glass ball which shatters when dropped. Just as a rubber ball rebounds without any permanent change to its inner composition, the play of life does not touch your inner being. You can gain the stability and strength to overcome high blood pressure.

You will see that hypertension is a disease of the body that can be overcome by mental strength. You will understand how you have been responsible for your illness and how to find a way out of this predicament. Cease to identify yourself with the objects around you and increase and cultivate your awareness of life to escape the effects of suffering and unhappiness, whether mental or physical.

78

Asana and Pranayama

Yoga includes a vast number of techniques which were designed to help the individual attain perfect health, and have been tried and tested for over 5,000 years. When you practise these techniques daily, you will regain your birthright, a healthy body and mind and thus will be able to enjoy life more. The aim of yoga is purely practical, to change your lifestyle so that you get more out of life.

Regular practice is essential. In endeavouring to reverse hypertension which has resulted from many years of tension and inadequate lifestyle, you must use a determined effort of willpower to achieve healing results. Sometimes it is like trying to push water uphill. This is not an impossible feat if you have the correct equipment such as a pump, but if you are not regular in your efforts, the water will quickly run back down and you will have to start all over again. With consistent effort, however, you can keep the water moving in the direction you desire, and eventually get it to where you want it. Then you can rest.

To cure yourself you must really want this. You have to do the work, no one else will do it for you and now is the time to start. At the same time you must have patience and perseverance and not be in a hurry. A good allegory of this is growing a plant. If you continually dig up the seed to see if it is growing, it will die. You should just carefully water it and care for the soil, and it will grow well.

We have devised a program of asana, pranayama and meditation techniques which is designed to give the seed of good health the best soil to grow in. Incorporate these practices into your day. They are safe, sure and steady in bringing about a complete change in the structure of your body and mind, so that rebalance and dynamism result.

These yogic practices lift you up so that you are no longer at the mercy of forces outside of yourself and beyond your control. Yoga allows you to gain this control. Try it and see; the surest sign of success is when your blood pressure goes down.

Asana

Asana means 'a steady and comfortable posture'. These are physical postures, both static and dynamic, which are designed to relax and strengthen the body and mind. They are not gymnastic exercises requiring strain and effort or muscle development, but afford relaxation, mobilize pranic energy and help you to gain more out of meditation. You should, therefore, not see asana as mere physical postures but as states of being, for their correct performance requires participation of one's whole being.

Asana require effortless effort in their performance. When practised correctly in conjunction with mental concentration and breath awareness they will allow you to achieve a state of integration or homeostasis, which indicates that the mechanism ensuring equilibrium of body and mind functions faultlessly. On the other hand, the wrong kind of exercise such as muscle building exercises can cause or aggravate hypertension. This kind of exercise gives emphasis purely on the physical side, ignoring the mental aspect, and thus leads to disharmony between mind and body and eventually to disease.

According to T. Pasek and Professor W. Romanowski from the Department of Physiology at the Academy of Physical Education, Poland: "The fundamental importance of psychic equilibrium for perfect health and physical efficiency is more and more appreciated by a wide circle of specialists in physical education. Investigators endeavour to find systems of physical education which, apart from training motor efficiency, will ensure psychic health... They turn therefore to the Oriental cultures, and primarily to the Yoga of India, to find educational systems that restore both psychic and physical equilibrium."[11]

Heavy physical exercises strain and tire the body, rather than giving energy. The muscles grow larger (hypertrophy) and consequently use up more oxygen. When the oxygen stores become depleted due to tension, heavy exercise, etc., the lactate level builds up and in higher amounts due to increased muscle bulk. This leads to exhaustion and subsequently to physical disease.

Asanas do not add to the muscle bulk but increase the efficiency and strength, for example, by aiding in the removal of lactic acid. They rest the body and facilitate oxygen utilization, which in itself prevents lactate formation, at the same time allowing more work to be carried out because oxygen gives more energy and strength through the oxidation of glucose (blood sugar).

Pasek and Romanowski state: "The essence of most physical exercises in yoga is relaxation/concentration gymnastics with the predominance of static (motionless) elements. These consist of assuming certain postures and using slackened breathing techniques. These exercises are coordinated with an imposed slackened breathing rhythm. They are performed in a state of absolute tranquility and with relaxed musculature; these are the indispensable conditions for simultaneous concentration."[12]

By maintaining a static asana, the body becomes dynamic and has time to readjust itself, be stretched, massaged, soothed, unknotted and relaxed. Asanas point out our deficiencies by the amount of discomfort we feel as we perform them. Tension produces discomfort in our usual waking lives, but during practice of asana, we feel the tightness and pain associated with tension as a real thing. It hurts! So it takes a little time to remove these tensions gradually and systematically, and bring relaxation of the muscles. Then we will be pain free and experience no discomfort.

Asanas also remove emotional and mental tension. The intensity of emotional states associated with our internal and external experience is reduced. The motor reactions associated with these states become far less violent. The cognitive (sensory awareness) and motor functions of the brain are soothed and integrated.

Pasek, Romanowski, et al. of Poland, and Vinekar of India, have conducted research and experiments which point to increased input to the brain from the various sensory receptors during asana practice. This occurs because of increased pressure on particular muscle and organ groups, while the muscles remain relaxed.[13,14] At the same time there is increased blood flow and oxygen to the brain, liver and other organs combined with excitation of certain centres within the brain through mental concentration. This increases tissue health through a massaging effect on the muscles and external organs affected; stimulation of the brain registering relaxation and removal of tension; and increase of prana in the pranic body, all adding up to increasing health. After some time, there is the development of a new pattern in the lower centres of the brain harmoniously integrated with the higher cortex, and conducive to good health. This is the important difference between yoga and ordinary exercise.

T. Pasek and Professor Romanowski have used physiological, biological and psychological methods in their tests. Their findings confirm that with systematic use of asana, better autonomic patterns, control and coordination evolve in the lower brain. This improves integration of brain functions, and emotional equilibrium and control are established to an extent not found in conventional physical cultures.

The work of T. Pasek, K.S. Gopal and others has supported the use of asana in diseases such as hypertension, and has shown that those people who use asana regularly are more relaxed than those who have never practised them before or who have just commenced yoga training.[15]

Gopal has linked his work with blood pressure studies, finding in favour of asana. He says that the hypometabolic state induced by asana and pranayama (reduced cell work and cell fatigue) and the resultant mental quietude are most beneficial in the treatment of hypertension. To test this, he carried out the following experiment:

1. *Aim*: To compare two groups of people practising asana; one group who have practised regularly for a period of six months and the other who were untrained. The subjects were connected to an EEG, and recordings were also made of peripheral blood flow and respiration.

2. *Experiment*: Subjects performed the following asana while the data was being recorded: vajrasana, shashankasana, sirshasana, shavasana, sarvangasana, vipareeta karani mudra, ardha matsyendrasana and setubandhasana.

3. *Results*: In untrained people, the degree of muscle relaxation was less than in the trained group, though both groups experienced maximum relaxation in shavasana, indicating that shavasana is better for hypertension. Also, in shavasana the heart rate and respiratory rates were least, while peripheral blood flow was at a maximum. In the trained group, heart rate and respiration were slower than in the untrained and the peripheral blood flow was greater. This indicates that the regular practice of asana increases the individual's ability to relax and lowers blood pressure by reducing the peripheral resistance. There was also increased alpha rhythm from the brain, correlating with relaxation of the nervous system.

In all the asana, the trained group needed less oxygen and gave out less carbon dioxide than the untrained group, showing that there was less effort involved and less metabolic activity. This indicates a deeper state of rest and relaxation. R. Wallace and H. Benson have reported that there is a reduction of the sympathetic nervous stimulation in all trained meditators, resulting in decreased peripheral resistance and thus, increased peripheral blood flow.[16] This agrees with Gopal's work.

Conclusion

Gopal has reported on shavasana that: "The electrical activity, heart rate and respiratory rate are minimal, and that peripheral blood flow is almost maximal. This represents a completely relaxed state of body and mind, and as such, is recommended for the treatment of hypertension."[17]

It has been shown that many diseases are linked with a crooked spine. If the spine is not straight, the energy from the brain is disturbed by pressure applied on the nerves from the spinal vertebral column. Experiments have shown that illness causes the spine to become crooked and that the crooked spine further predisposes to illness. For example:

• A lesion at the level of the third and fourth thoracic vertebrae can lead to heart trouble and asthma.
• A lesion at the level of the fifth to ninth thoracic vertebrae can cause digestive disease.
• A warp in the seventh cervical or fifth thoracic vertebrae has been correlated with nervous and mental disorders.

Misaligned vertebrae can press on the nerves as they emerge from the spinal cord through the spinal column and either block the flow of impulses or increase it by irritating the nerve roots. In either case, disordered function of the organs can occur. Asana prevent this by straightening the spinal column. The asana realign the individual bones and discs of cartilage and encourage blood flow to nourish the spinal cord and associated nerve plexes.

Asana also recondition the body in many other ways. During asana practice, the massage of the internal organs helps to squeeze out stale blood, allowing the flow of fresh blood into the tissues. Asana rebalance the endocrine glands, preventing the adrenal overactivity caused by instability of the nervous system. When the endocrine glands are reintegrated, the body's metabolism is optimal.

84

Through their effect on the endocrine glands and spine, asana stimulate and help to rebalance the chakras. The whole body is made to pulsate synchronously with life-giving prana. Each cell has its own consciousness which is brought back into harmony with the consciousness of every other cell so that the body attains a new and vital rhythm.

Asana are also spiritual exercises comprising the third step in the eightfold path of Patanjali's raja yoga system. They are the first step on the royal path to highest consciousness and, of course, any process leading to higher awareness removes hypertension.

Pranayama

Prana is the vital force which pervades the whole cosmos. It is in all things and is the bioenergy that activates the human organism; the life within the seed that makes it grow. It is closely related to the air we breathe, which is our main source of prana. However, air is only the physical vehicle to be used and manipulated in the process of extraction of prana. Prana links body and mind, so that its control offers much in terms of helping hypertension.

Yama means 'control' and pranayama are that group of techniques that aims at stimulating or balancing the vital energy. They purify the pranic body and remove blocks, allowing energy to flow freely.

Prana is the energy used by psychic healers and 'faith' healers. It is said to have been photographed by Kirlian photography and is the subject of much research, especially in Russia and USA. The experiments suggest that when a person is sick, he emits a certain energy pattern from which it is possible to diagnose his state of health. It is also suggested that the colours of the electrical discharge indicate the emotions being experienced at that moment.

Kirlian photographs seem not to be of the actual aura, but possibly a reflection of the pranic body in the electrical field. Interesting research is coming from many quarters showing the effects on this field of disease, health, psychic healing, asana, pranayama and meditation. This is a promising new area for tomorrow.

The first objective evidence of the pranic body, or the 'aura' and the chakras, may have already been obtained by a UCLA (American) study assisted by an 'aura reader' named Dr Bruyere and incorporating a number of different measurements.

Kinesiologist, Valerie Hunt and her associates at UCLA utilize an electromyograph, which measures the steady, low-voltage wave forms representing the electrical activity in the muscles. The subjects were undergoing 'rolfing', a form of structural integration using manipulation and massage of the fascia designed to break up deep muscle tension and rigidity. Electrodes were attached to eight traditional chakra locations and acupuncture sites such as the eyebrow centre (*ajna chakra*), the crown of the head (*sahasrara chakra*), *anahata chakra* behind the heart and so on. While massage was in progress the EMG recorded the changes on one track of a two-track tape recorder while simultaneously Bruyere recorded on the audio track a description of the colour, size and activity of the auric field of the subjects and rolfers. Using a second microphone, subjects described their spontaneous experience and images during rolfing.

"It was quickly evident that the distinctive wave forms on the oscilloscope correlated with the colours reported by the sensitive.

'The possible interpretations are staggering,' Hunt acknowledged, adding that these radiations had been taken directly from the body surface, 'quantitatively measured in a natural state... isolated by scientifically accepted data-reduction procedures.'

Whether by wave form, Fourier-frequency analysis or by Sonagram, the data produced the same results and consistently correlated with the reader's colour label."[18]

Rumanian scientists have developed a method of body scanning they call electronography.[19] It is similar to the Kirlian method but is more sophisticated, using a variety of recording devices ranging from black-and-white photography to coloured videotapes. These images are produced by varying an electromagnetic field generated by a unique high voltage field. More than 6,000 people have undergone electronography at the Labour Protection and Hygiene Centre in Bucharest and experimental studies in cancer have revealed that it is possible to detect differences between healthy and sick tissues. The light intensity varies, for example, between dark for inflammation to light for cancer. Using this 'auric diagnosis' will open extensive areas in preventive and therapeutic medicine. By detecting subtle changes in the body fields in a regular medical checkup, we can see slight abnormalities in pattern, field and intensity, in order to prevent future disease from occurring.

The findings of these experiments support the claims of yogis that a subtle energy sheath exists as a frame of reference beyond the visible spectrum, organizing and vitalizing the physical body. Through yogic training we can become aware of this pranic sheath and manipulate prana for our better health, controlling our emotional and mental states as well as the resilience and plasticity of the tissues in the physical body. Asana remove the encoded tension gradually, painlessly and systematically, by stretching out the 'wrinkles' in the muscles while allowing us to manipulate our nervous system via relaxed concentration. They also raise our levels of prana.

Pranayama, too, increases the content of prana in the body, and the smoothness and uniformity of the energy field around the body. Pranayama allows us to fill the body with prana so that it flows like liquid into all the pores of the skin, filling up any defects in the aura and reviving and revitalizing all the organs of the body. The body soaks up this energy like a sponge and uses this prana to power all the vital processes.

The breath and the heart are linked together. When we speed up our breathing, we speed up our heart. This can be demonstrated by the following experiment. Sit in a comfortable position and hold the pulse of the left wrist with the right first two fingers. For between five and ten minutes count five beats of the pulse on inhalation and five on exhalation. The pulse will be seen to slow and you will experience the feeling of relaxation.

This exercise demonstrates that the mind is also linked to the breath and heart. When you are anxious the heart and breath speed up; when you are relaxed heart and breath slow down. The control of the breath can therefore influence the heart and help to relieve hypertension.

Swami Kuvalyananda at Kaivalyadhama, near Bombay in India, has shown that pranayama relaxes the metabolic processes by increasing the utilization of oxygen in the tissues. With each breath there is increased oxygen consumption and carbon dioxide expulsion, indicating that the cells are working better and purifying themselves more thoroughly. Overall, there is a general decrease in oxygen intake, but an increase in how efficiently it is used. This is a hypometabolic state, conducive to the lowering of blood pressure. The body extracts more energy from the oxygen it uses thereby spending less energy trying to get oxygen to the tissues. The result is that there is more energy for healing and better living.

How pranayama works

Normally the respiratory and cardiovascular systems (lungs, heart and blood vessels) work automatically, although they can be consciously governed with willpower and awareness. In the link between heart and lungs, the nervous system plays a most important part in monitoring blood pressure and blood chemistry to ensure that everything is functioning smoothly. Any changes are detected by sensitive baro-receptors for pressure, and chemoreceptors for detecting the levels of oxygen and carbon dioxide. When a change is required, signals are sent through the sympathetic or parasympathetic nervous systems instructing to either speed up or slow down the lungs and heart, and to adjust the peripheral resistance.

The following increase the rate of breathing, heart beat and blood pressure: pain, unpleasant stimuli, fall in peripheral blood pressure, decrease in oxygen concentration, and tension.

The following decrease the rate of breathing, heartbeat and blood pressure: warmth, pleasant stimuli, massage, hot baths, most asanas, increased arterial oxygen (via pranayama) and relaxation.

So we see that pranayama, by raising the oxygen concentration, decreases the blood pressure in the fastest and most efficient way. Some pranayama, such as ujjayi and nadi shodhana also reduce the pressure by directly cutting the activity of the sympathetic nervous system.

Pranayama has the following effects:

1. The mind is relaxed, decreasing sympathetic arousal.
2. The oxygen level of the blood increases and the efficiency of oxygen utilization by the tissues is maximized leading to deeper relaxation and more energy.
3. The carbon in the system slowly increases and this has the effect of strengthening the nervous system leading to better overall health.

Hence, pranayama is not just a breathing exercise. Through pranayama we can influence the basic cellular metabolism and the structure of the nervous system and, in so doing, increase or decrease the energy until it is balanced. In the treatment of hypertension the following pranayama are used:

- Ujjayi to relax the body energy flow.
- Nadi shodhana to balance the energy flow.

Ujjayi also acts directly on the carotid sinuses which are the pressure receptors in the neck. When pressure is greater, the carotid sinuses cause the heart rate to slow in order to reduce the blood pressure. Ujjayi exerts a gentle pressure on these receptors, so that the blood pressure falls to low levels associated with relaxation. Ujjayi directs pranic flow towards the medulla oblongata of the spinal cord at the top of the neck. This is the area from which stem many parasympathetic nerves, so that by stimulation of the parasympathetic nervous system the autonomic nervous system can be rebalanced, enhancing further reduction of blood pressure. Blood pressure stability is achieved through relaxation of nerve centres in the medulla which control the calibre of the blood vessels. The blood vessels become less constricted so that blood flows through under less pressure.

Abdominal or 'yogic' breathing has been tested by Dr Motoyama, Director of the International Association for Religion and Parapsychology in Japan. He showed that contraction and release of the abdominal muscles heightens mental and physical vitality. The plethsymograph of subjects practising deep abdominal breathing in an erect sitting position indicates an improvement in overall blood circulation.

EEG tracings of brain waves during abdominal breathing show an increase in alpha waves, indicating deep relaxation of the nervous system in this practice.

Motoyama states: "Pranayama is also seemingly able to hinder the occurrence of angina pectoris. Certain hospitals have been recommending their heart patients, particularly with angina pectoris, to begin abdominal breathing when they feel an attack coming on. The reports are that this practice has been successful and that it is being continued."[20]

Combined techniques

The techniques of yoga have a definite place in the treatment of hypertension. They are used to fill in the gaps left by modern science. Medicine reduces blood pressure in the acute situation and yoga removes it in the long term preventing further recurrence and the often catastrophic sequel to prolonged hypertension.

Much evidence exists that yoga can be utilized in the treatment of hypertension as a means to gradually reduce and then eliminate the use of drugs.

The Patanjali Yoga Institute (Hyderabad, India) tested a series of asana and pranayama used by a group of patients with essential hypertension.[21] Almost all patients had been on anti-hypertensive medication and a salt-free diet. These had been useful in preventing major complications of the disease, so that their hearts and blood vessels were still functioning well.

After clinical assessment the patients commenced the asana and pranayama and their blood pressures were measured at intervals throughout the day, before and after the practices. At the same time the drugs were tapered off, although if the patient did not respond adequately, ayurvedic medicines were used as well. (Ayurveda is the ancient system of medicine in India, closely aligned with yoga.)

Of the cases reported, the first is that of a fifty-five year old man being treated with Reserpine, a most powerful anti-hypertensive drug, over a five year period. He started practising yoga and in only five days his blood pressure had reduced so much that he could stop the drug. After this there was a steady decline in blood pressure from the initial pre-treatment level of 230/120 mm Hg to a normal pressure of 130/80 mm Hg. He returned home and continued with yoga. His blood pressure has remained normal and his general health is good.

Another example is that of a woman aged forty-eight who was not using any drugs or salt restriction. Her initial blood pressure was 190/104 mm Hg. The practice of yoga alone brought it down to 140/90 mm Hg. Thereafter she was given ayurvedic drugs and the pressure came down to 110/70 mm Hg.

K.K. Datey BA, MD, FICA (USA), FRCP (Lond.) et al., working in K.E.M. Hospital, Bombay, India, has used a combination of shavasana and abdominal breathing in treating hypertension. Datey states: "The anti-hypertensive drugs available so far are by no means ideal and have many disadvantages. Any other method for reducing blood pressure, therefore, is most welcome... In this connection, we present a new approach – management of hypertension with shavasana, a yogic exercise."[22]

91

Most of Datey's patients had been under observation for two years while their drug therapy was being stabilized. Any attempts at reducing the drug dosage had led to an increase in blood pressure. Most of the patients also had one or more of the following symptoms: giddiness, headache, chest pain (a sign of heart disease), palpitations, breathlessness on exertion, insomnia, irritability and nervousness.

They were then taught shavasana. This yogic technique is fully explained in the practice section and involves lying on the back and relaxing the whole body whilst concentrating on abdominal breathing. The whole exercise takes about thirty minutes and its technique is quite simple. Actually, the ashrams inspired by Swami Satyananda Saraswati teach a similar but much more powerful yogic technique known as yoga nidra.

Datey's experiment showed significant reduction in drug dosage and blood pressure in more than half the patients. Of the other half, those who had evidence of hardening of the arteries showed no response, demonstrating the importance of early treatment before the vicious circle has cemented. A significant proportion of the remainder had not done the exercise properly. When they were finally convinced of the necessity of correctness and regularity, they too showed improvement.

The overall majority of patients showed improvement in symptoms. Headache, nervousness, giddiness, irritability and sleeplessness had disappeared in almost all. The other symptoms were lessened and most of the patients felt a general sense of wellbeing after performing shavasana.

Datey stated: "The exercise is easy to perform, has no side-effects and needs no equipment. There was symptomatic relief and a sense of wellbeing in the vast majority of patients. This therapy opens up a new avenue for the treatment of hypertension."[23]

From this evidence it can be seen that yoga asana and pranayama have a lot to offer in the treatment of hypertension and the reduction or elimination of anti-hypertensive drugs.

It must be remembered that illnesses such as hypertension take a long time to manifest. For perhaps years, unconscious forces have been moulding the body and brain circuitry to produce the necessary pathways for sympathetic hyperactivity. Hence it cannot be expected of any system that it produces immediate cure or any other miracle.

Yoga will produce a reduction in symptoms very quickly but it takes time for all of the neurones in the brain to be restored and for the body to change. However, while this is going on, yoga offers you freedom from stresses and from the symptoms themselves.

Yogic Way of Life

When you come to understand your place in the universal flow of things through the practice of meditation, your life takes on a new meaning. You find a great deal of peace and happiness inside and this lasts throughout the day giving you fulfilment and a new understanding of yourself and the meaning life has for you. This is the surest way to reverse the whole of that lifestyle which has led to hypertension. It is achieved through yoga.

The fact that you have hypertension indicates that there are defects in the way you are living. To overcome these defects you will slowly have to change. The basic aspects of your life are changed first and the other points change in their time. Then everything falls into place.

The yogic lifestyle is a natural one in accordance with the natural laws around us. It is important to follow these laws in order to be free from disease and to maintain good health. We become integrated people, at one with ourselves and with the world. We cannot escape from this earth on which we are born and from which our bodies are made. It is for this reason that yoga has propounded scientific laws based on centuries of experience, which only recently have been highlighted through modern science.

Two important aspects of our lifestyle are our sleeping and eating habits. It is these that we will discuss in this chapter on lifestyle.

Sleep patterns

"Early to bed, early to rise, makes you healthy, wealthy and wise." This is an old recipe for good health that has at its core much wisdom. It is the ancient formula which is being proven today through scientific research and which has been propounded by yogis for thousands of years. Scientists have found that the most refreshing and restful sleep comes in the first hours of sleep. By going to bed early we gain more benefit from each hour of slumber, because this then allows us to get up early and thereby take advantage of the natural rhythms of our body and thereby improve the quality and quantity of our waking hours by being more alert, active and dynamic.

Stress disrupts·the natural biorhythms and disturbs our waking, dreaming and sleeping hours. This is indicated by the number of sleeping pills on the market and the number of people who take them. When we are awake, stress causes us to feel anxious, exhausted, easily aggravated and therefore limits our natural potential and effectiveness. In sleep, tension causes nightmares and restlessness. People under stress have difficulty in falling asleep and waking up and thus they get out of bed feeling tired and unrefreshed. Many people complain to their doctors that they feel too tired during the day to work effectively or enjoy life.

Pills to cure sleep problems are not only ineffective but harmful and compound the problems causing hypertension. Tranquilizers cut out the dream phase of sleep which is so important for release of tension. This results in increased fatigue during the day, more tension at night and the need for more pills. Once begun, if we stop using sleeping pills the suppressed dream mechanism is overactivated, causing nightmares that frighten the patient back to his bottle of pills. Thus the vicious circle continues.

Sleep has four basic stages which shade progressively into deepening consciousness. During the period of sleep, there are five or six occasions when we emerge from the deeper phases into a lighter state of consciousness, rapid

95

eye movement (REM) sleep. At this time, although the muscles of the body remain totally relaxed, there is disturbed breathing and flickering of the eyelids. If the person is awakened during this phase, he reports that he was dreaming. If an electroencephalograph (brain wave graph) is taken, the tracing is similar to that taken during the waking state. Experiments have shown that if people are prevented from having this dream sleep, they become irritable during the day. Then when they are allowed to sleep through, they have many more episodes of the rapid eye movement stage and their irritability settles. It seems that dreams are necessary for emotional wellbeing, so we can imagine the adverse effects of long-standing intake of sleeping pills, which suppress dreaming.

Early morning awakening has been recommended since time immemorial. The time between 4 a.m. and 6 a.m. is known by the yogis as *brahmamuhurta*, the hours of Brahma the creator and is held to be the best time for spiritual practice. At this time, the mental and spiritual energies are at their highest. The body and mind are prepared to begin the day in the most efficient way. The longer we sleep after this, the harder it is to get out of bed. We sink into the trough that follows the crest of every wave.

Experiments on rats by Dr Barry Jacobs at the Stanford Medical School have shown that during the daydreaming is inhibited by the hormone serotonin, which is secreted from the pineal gland. Serotonin reaches maximum concentration in the body around six in the morning, indicating that the body is primed for active waking at that time.

Melatonin is another hormone which is secreted by the pineal gland at night. It is thought to inhibit sexual energy and its secretion stops at around 4 a.m. Thus from this time on, the vital energy that powers the sex drive and other activity is in action.

Interlocked with the above cycles is the production of ACTH by the pituitary gland. ACTH is the messenger hormone that stimulates the adrenal glands to secrete cortisone which releases sugar and energy for use in the body and helps adaptation to stress. The maximum secretion of ACTH also occurs at 4 a.m. By getting up at this time we begin the day on the crest of an energy wave, making the best of the body's resources while they are at their peak.

If we get up at 4 a.m. we can use this energy for mental benefit and spiritual enhancement during the practice of yoga. We can turn sexual energy into a life-giving force called ojas. This does not mean that we become celibate or feel like giving up sexual activity, just the reverse happens. Sexual activity is balanced and is used for all areas of physical, emotional, mental and spiritual wellbeing. This is part of the science of tantra; an ancient system where nothing is suppressed and everything is used. By getting up early in the morning and doing our yoga practice, we not only conserve energy, but we can increase it so that life becomes more vibrant and joyful.

Getting up early in the morning also eliminates insomnia, because it is easier to get to sleep when we have risen so early. We are pleasantly relaxed and feel that the day has been full. This produces a feeling of warm satisfaction and sleep fulfils its natural and rest-providing function.

If we ignore the benefits of brahmamuhurta, we are more prone to stress and high blood pressure. By getting up early, we assist the process of eliminating hypertension and improving the health. Make early rising a part of your life and experience the full implications of bringing your life back into harmony with the flow of natural rhythms and cycles of the universe.

Eating habits

This is an important aspect in the management of high blood pressure. Faulty diet is considered by some to be a major cause of hypertension. When you consider how much the average person loads into his stomach and how much of what he eats is harmful to his health, then you will not be surprised that there is so much hypertension and constipation in our community. A reduction in salt intake alone will reduce blood pressure.

All people with hypertension must reduce their intake of salt to the barest minimum. This means no salt added while cooking food and no table salt added after preparation. This is only a temporary step while you are reducing blood pressure; when it is normal again, salt can again be gradually added, but henceforth only in moderate amounts. Actually, with time, a saltless diet can be as enjoyable as one with salt. After all, most people add salt only because of habit; there are many herbs and spices that we can substitute.

Obesity is an inefficient way for a body to move around in this world and must also be reduced. Overweight makes extra work for all our organs and puts a load on all body systems. People who are carrying extra weight may become used to their condition, but just the same the extra work incurred by the body shortens the lifespan and the quality of life itself. When obesity is added to hypertension, the condition can be quite dangerous.

It has been proven that with the aid of proper eating habits, it is possible to extend one's lifespan. There exist some people, for instance the Hunzas, who have a much longer lifespan than others. In general such people live in tune with nature and their diet is a natural one.

Dr David Davies, a professor at London University, reported on the residents of the Vilacamba Valley in Ecuador after a field trip in 1973. He stated that: "Their diet is mainly vegetarian, with oranges, bananas, apples and lots of vegetables. They eat only an ounce of meat a week and virtually no animal fat."[24] One farmer was energetically working in his field at the age of 147.

The *National Geographic* (January 1973) reports: "Dr Guillermo Vela of Quito found a strikingly low consumption of calories among the people of Vilacamba. The average diet contained only 1200 calories. The daily protein was 35 to 38 grams, of fat only 12 to 19 grams and 200 to 260 grams of carbohydrate completed the diet. Protein and fat were largely of vegetable origin, with only a few grams of protein daily from animal sources. Compare this with the 2500–5000 calories per day in the average western diet. "Needless to say Dr Vela saw no obesity among the elderly in Vilacamba and it does not occur in the Hunzas; neither were there signs of malnutrition."

This diet sounds very much like the ashram diet. On a simple yet complete diet of approximately 1500 calories per day the swamis of the ashram rise at three o'clock and go to bed no earlier than nine. This makes an average work day of sixteen to eighteen hours a day. The ashram diet is rice, vegetables, split peas or lentils (dahl), whole wheat unleavened bread (chappatis) and fruit and green salad from time to time. On this the health of every person in the ashram has been increased to optimum level.

On a trial conducted by the IYFM Research Coordinating Centre at the Bihar School of Yoga, the blood pressures of the residents of the ashram were measured. The figures are only preliminary and have yet to be put to more complete and exacting trial. However, they do suggest the benefits of a sensible diet, yoga and living the natural way of life.

The people in the ashram were divided into three groups:
Group 1: Swamis who had lived in the ashram for more than a year.
Group 2: Swamis who had lived in the ashram for less than a year.
Group 3: Visitors to the ashram, many of whom had been on the average western meat diet before arriving.
On this basis the blood pressures were averaged as follows:
Group 1: 100.50 mm Hg
Group 2: 110.60 mm Hg
Group 3: 120.80 mm Hg

The fact that the blood pressures are so low in a group of people all sharing the same environment suggests that the sympathetic activity is very low. This is probably because the yogic way of life is in tune with nature, in terms of attitude, activity and eating habits.

99

According to the teachings of yoga, the digestive system is ruled by manipura chakra, which is also the pranic generator of the digestive fire. If we eat heavy meals, or poorly cooked ones or poor quality food, we decrease the amount of prana in the body. Thus the whole organism is devitalized and our resistance to disease is lowered.

Poor quality food tastes bad. Artificially made and preserved foods or food prepared without care and that intangible quality called 'love' just do not taste as good as high quality, simple foods which are eaten in a relaxed and congenial setting. Prana is added to the food through the hands which are the organs of expression of the heart. Hands are a means of expressing our inner feelings in the outer world. They transmit prana in the case of the person who is giving and they absorb prana in the case of the person who cooks with a selfish or otherwise negative attitude.

By taking care of our diet and ensuring consistency in this area of our lives, it is inevitable that we increase our prana and health. One more area of our lives is made healthy and ordered. We gradually lift ourselves out of the mire and darkness of hypertension and into the light of good health. All the other areas of our life naturally fall into their correct perspective and our wellbeing increases.

Relaxation and Awareness

Every yogic practice is based on these two simple and straightforward aspects of human existence: relaxation and awareness. No matter how high or difficult the technique, these two elements are at its base and core. Relaxed awareness is the key to aware relaxation, the cure for the condition of hypertension.

The relaxed mind is an alert mind, ever ready to deal with the problem of hypertension. In this state we can:

• prevent the occurrence of new problems and disturbances
• exhaust the conscious problems of which you are aware
• discover and eradicate subconscious problems.

The more you discover in your conscious mind, the more easily you will be able to bring subconscious disturbances to the surface. These are the complexes which are deep in the mind and make their presence felt in the form of depression or fear, without knowing their cause.

These three processes occur simultaneously and though there are many techniques, all depend on relaxation with awareness. Mental problems can only be removed when the mind relaxes. This initiates a virtuous circle of: relaxation... bringing the removal of mental problems... leading to deeper relaxation. You will understand this better when you experience it for yourself.

When you have cultivated a relaxed state of mind, you have conscious control and can command every part of your body to let its tensions go. You will only need a little practice of yoga nidra or other forms of meditation to relax the body totally. When you can do this, you will be able consciously to relax your blood vessels so that they can be dilated and constricted at will. The ability to relax decreases the blood pressure.

Yogic techniques allow you to go within yourself and disconnect from the physical body, experiencing a state of pure awareness. This quietens the activity of the mind and cerebral cortex of the brain, which in time quietens the whole body. It shuts off the worrying process enabling the 'higher' intellectual regions of the nervous system to integrate with the 'lower' feeling regions. Intuitive understanding then arises instantly and spontaneously.

Brain wave demonstration
Integration of brain functions has been reported by researchers experimenting with meditators, who base their results on brain wave measurements. There are four main types of waves:

1. *Beta waves* are the patterns that predominate during our everyday, wakeful state. They are related to external activities – extroversion. When we engage the brain in rational thinking, when we are tense, anxious or just in a 'normal' frame of mind, beta waves predominate in our brains and on the EEG (electroencephalograph). These waves are small, coming faster than thirteen cycles per second.

2. *Alpha waves* are emitted during milder states of meditation. They are related to relaxed awareness, to passivity and to a non-anxious, tension-free state. They are also related to states of creativity so that during these periods they are the dominant wave form. Alpha waves are slightly larger than beta waves and come somewhere between eight and thirteen times per second.

3. *Theta waves* are emitted during dreaming and are associated with the subconscious mind. Theta waves

predominate also in deeper states of meditation, intense creativity, ecstasy and receptivity to ESP. Children may emit this wave in their waking state, though this is rare in adults. The frequency range of this wave is from four to seven cycles per second.

4. *Delta waves* are large, slow waves of less than four per second. They predominate in dreamless sleep, but have also been recorded in deep states of meditation.

Through the practices of yoga the brain is systematically reorganized into a healthier and better coordinated state. Over time, the alpha and theta content of the brain waves increases which means that the nervous system is 'beating' more strongly and slowly; the state associated with serenity, creativity, enhanced receptivity and joy. Yoga soothes the autonomic nervous system, thereby eradicating increased blood pressure.

Through yoga, the brain and mind are rested from the constant stream of disturbing sensory input from outside and thus we become aware of our own inner being.

Biofeedback demonstration

Biofeedback is a training system which sometimes uses an EEG machine to determine when the subject is producing mainly alpha waves and thus help him recognize and control relaxed states of mind. The technique itself uses electronic machines to detect changes in the body. When the desired change is achieved, the machine registers this by a tone signal or a flashing light. In this way it feeds back information that the person has manipulated his body in the correct way. The usual aim is for him to gain conscious control over actions of his body which are usually not voluntary, such as the local skin temperature, blood pressure or, as in this case, the brain rhythms.

In biofeedback we induce a state of relaxed awareness (the alpha state) in order to learn how to direct processes that were once thought to be automatic and beyond the influence of the will. In doing this, great importance is given to the techniques of visualization and one-pointedness of mind. These techniques are developed by yoga and bring about the same control of body and mind, but without the need for machines.

Examples of biofeedback technique

This method of directing the involuntary functions of the body through the mind has been used successfully in the treatment of hypertension and heart disease, incorporating the techniques of awareness and relaxation.

In an experiment by Dr David Shapiro of the Harvard Medical School, a subject is placed in a cubicle controlled for light and sound.[25] He is seated with a cuff of a sphygmomanometer (machine that measures blood pressure) around his arm and a microphone in the cuff of the machine to amplify the sound of the pulse beat at the elbow. The sound makes the patient aware of his blood pressure and he learns to adjust it. These findings have been reproduced in other experiments such as those by Jasper Brener et al., at the University of Tennessee.[26]

Aimee Christy and John Vitale of the San Francisco Veterans' Administration Hospital report that biofeedback training has proven to be successful in two cases of labile hypertension.[27]

Dr Herbert Benson of Harvard University has helped five of his patients to reduce their blood pressure with biofeedback training. He reports: "...Nevertheless, to generalize this training and keep blood pressure down at home and at the office, may require some revision of behaviour and even re-evaluation of lifestyle, as well as some professional behaviour therapy."[28]

The revision of lifestyle is offered by yoga and by living in a healthy natural way. The combination of biofeedback and yoga appears even more promising when we consider the results of experimentation on meditation, asanas and pranayama. The combination of such practices provides a potent battery of methods which, when used under close

104

supervision, will give the healer a wide range of techniques to remove not only the patient's symptoms and suffering, but to get at the root of the cause.

The number of people researching this field is growing and the fact that so many eminent scientists are seriously investigating the process suggests that there is something valuable in this form of treatment. We have established the fact that a person can regulate his own blood pressure and heartbeat through mental discipline alone. This points to the day when biofeedback will be used as an integral part of widespread treatment programs.

A study conducted by Dr Engle at Baltimore City Hospital, USA, has already used biofeedback for heart disease as follows:[29]

1. *Aim*: To find if eight subjects could learn to control dangerous irregularities in their heartbeat by the use of mental concentration and discipline. The irregularity used in this experiment was premature ventricular contractions which are associated with an increased incidence of sudden death.

2. *Method*: In a dark and windowless laboratory, the patient lay comfortably on a hospital bed connected up to a cardiotachometer, which converts the heartbeat into electric signals. These signals were fed into a computer, analyzed and translated into red, yellow and green lights which showed on a panel at the foot of the bed. The patient was told to 'drive' his heartbeat. He was to slow his heart when he saw the red light and to speed it when he saw the green light. The aim was to keep the heart beating at a safe and steady rhythm, indicated by the yellow light.

3. *Results*: Using biofeedback signals, the patient first learns to speed the heart, then slow it, then finally it keep it within the narrow limits of normal.

4. *Conclusion*: People can learn to control and regulate potentially dangerous cardiac arrhythmias solely through the power of the mind.

Gay Luce and Eric Peper, reviewing biofeedback research for the New York Times Magazine, emphasize: "Training may be fundamentally tedious and may require a long time, but unlike drugs, it gives the person a sense of mastery over his own body. One of the women in Dr Engel's group was elated when she could report that she no longer had dizzy spells or thumping heart because of her new ability to cope with the symptoms."[30]

Perhaps the most exciting part of this study is to see what happens when the patient is disconnected from the training equipment and sent home to fend for himself. After sufficient training he can regulate his heartbeat without the need of artificial feedback. One of the eight patients has sustained her normal rate for almost two years, reporting that she is able to detect and modify her irregular heartbeat any time. Three others have had similar results outside the laboratory. Most of these patients cannot describe just how they accomplish their cardiac control, although one man imagines he is pushing his heart to the left and one woman imagines she is swinging it back and forth. Visualization is an important part of cure and this is intensified by the practice of yoga.

The use of yogic techniques ensure control in terms of mind and body. By employing meditative techniques along with biofeedback, increased relaxation and understanding are gained through direct experience of the mind. Meditation teaches what the mind is. Through concentration exercises it enables the subject to feel the interconnections between the voluntary nervous system and the autonomic nervous system. In this way balance and control of the body processes are achieved. The combination of yoga and biofeedback will prove to be a powerful method in the reduction of high blood pressure as well as in other forms of heart and circulatory disease.

We learn control of the brain waves through suggestion. We can also learn control of the brain in the same fashion that we learn anything else, through feedback from our environment (internal and external) via our senses and deeper intuition. The electronic biofeedback machine just augments the 2,000 or so organic biofeedback mechanisms that already exist within our bodies. The unconscious internal states are brought to external awareness.

It is possible through awareness of biofeedback signals to enhance healing of psychosomatic disorders. When we are aware of our body we can control its functions, such as dampening of sympathetic tone and the subsequent decrease of peripheral resistance which lowers blood pressure. The alpha state of the brain can also be extended so that we go through life in a relaxed and creative state of mind free from the entanglement of attachments.

Application of biofeedback in the management of hypertension has been reported by Dr C. H. Patel. Using a biofeedback device that measured 'relaxation,' sixteen in twenty people improved their hypertension and reduced their drug intake.

Patel states: "Yogic relaxation and biofeedback were used in the treatment of twenty patients with hypertension. As a result, anti-hypertensive therapy was stopped altogether in five patients and reduced by 33 percent to 60 percent in a further seven patients. Blood pressure control was better in four other patients, whilst the other four did not respond. Of these four, at least one had derived indirect benefit by the relief of migraine and depression. The results of this study promise a useful new approach to the treatment of hypertension.

The yogic technique Patel used was concentration on the breath. They could mentally repeat: 'relaxed... relaxed... relaxed' with every expiration (as a mantra). The concentration kept them mentally alert, but inwardly aware.[31]

Patients attended three times a week, for half an hour each time, over three months. During the entire time they were connected to the relaxometer which changed sympathetic activity into sound. The patient had to reduce the tone of the sound or top it.

Patel has worked out a treatment program consisting of:

1. Information about hypertension and the medicines used to treat it, information about biofeedback and research on psychological treatment of hypertension.
2. Individual instruction and training in yoga relaxation involving awareness of the body, the spontaneous breath and repetition of the word 'relaxed' at each expiration. During laboratory training the subject is connected to a skin resistance feedback machine, with the instruction to keep a low tone, that is a high resistance, denoting relaxation.
3. Instruction in the use of relaxation in everyday life and encouragement to have regular short periods of relaxation during the day. Other examples are to have a red sign on their watches to remind them to 'relax' each time they want to know the time of day. Others are told to recall the attitude of relaxation for a moment before answering the telephone.

Patel's results are very promising in all spheres and they demonstrate the exciting opportunities for humanity which can result from the marriage of the ancient science of yoga and modern technology. At present, as each new drug is developed and each new surgical procedure is created, the patient becomes more and more dependent on his doctor and loses his self-reliance. Biofeedback is the first technology to return to the patient responsibility for his own health. This process used the patient's own built-in self-regulating mechanism of which most people are completely unaware. This results in autonomy, independence and satisfaction in being able to govern his own body and heal himself of hypertension or any other illness.

Yoga and biofeedback begin the process of giving back a degree of responsibility to the patient. They have been shown to work in hypertension and other psychosomatic areas but their full potential has yet to be thoroughly developed. The day has dawned when doctors prescribe training such as yoga and biofeedback instead of drugs.

Until now, technology has limited man's personal capacities. However, biofeedback is an attempt to extend capacities using technology as a catalyst.

Yoga uses awareness, relaxation, visualization and willpower techniques found over thousands of years of experience to be most effective in remoulding body and mind. Asanas massage and tone the body organs and rebalance the endocrine-chakra pair; pranayama controls the life force and meditation plumbs the depths of the mind, awakening its inherent healing power to overcome hypertension. When yoga and biofeedback are used together, the process is made even more powerful. Biofeedback gives us instant awareness of the internal processes and how to govern them, and yoga gives us the techniques to do this and also to extend control and autonomy into every department of life.

Meditation

Meditation is a method of extending our ordinary consciousness and thereby discovering more about ourselves. When we gain this insight we can change our habits and our deeper, inner personality has a better chance to show through. Our whole life changes for the better. We remove problems from the past which are fermenting in the mind, changing shape, colour and intensity, but still lying there waiting to be resolved. These are the root problems that cause hypertension.

The many facets of meditation

Meditation is a technique of turning down the brilliance of the day so that the subtle sources of energy can be perceived within. Generally, because of the 'glare' of fast, tense modern living, we lose a lot of useful information coming in through the senses; this is a kind of mental 'squinting.' Meditation is a deliberate attempt to isolate ourselves from the flow of external 'reality' so that we remove the glare and have a chance to rest deeply and fully.

When we find a 'place' within where we can refresh ourselves, it becomes easier to handle external problems. We gain a new perspective on life so that these difficulties are seen as forces outside ourselves. Meditation allows us to objectify problems and to remove the subjective elements so that we can extricate ourselves from the web of emotional and mental tensions that is holding us fixed and rigid in our present predicament. Even hypertension becomes clearly visible as a situation that can be remedied.

Meditation is proving to be useful in all walks of life. It is especially helpful in alleviating illnesses such as hypertension. However, this is only the first step. Meditation has the power to unfold the latent potential in every human being, and modern research has proved conclusively that the benefits of meditation are of value to all people. Its success can be gauged by the increasing number of people absorbing meditation into their life pattern. Even the US Army, government institutions and high-ranking business executives are meditating.

Today we are seeing the emergence of meditation as a vital aspect of modern life. A vacuum which has existed in many of our lives has led to feelings of hopelessness, unhappiness and frustration. This vacuum is today being filled by a new sense of meaning gained from the ancient yogic techniques of meditation. As this vacuum is filled, the imbalance between man's inner and outer worlds is being redressed. Instead of constantly looking outside of himself for happiness, satisfaction and fulfilment, the meditator is discovering that the inner world is the source of sublime happiness and security. This realization can be used to cultivate a better outer world so that stress and tension can no longer impinge on inner life and create unhappiness, suffering and hypertension. This rebalance occurs in the body as equilibrium of the ida/pingala nadis; the sympathetic and parasympathetic nervous systems.

Effects on our daily lives

Research has shown that meditation has the following effects on our mind and daily life:

- Rebalances and stabilizes the nervous system. It encourages a natural and automatic response within the nervous system that counteracts and corrects the imbalances that occur through the day.

111

- Induces a deep state of rest which encourages the repair of those tissues damaged by hypertension and improves the health of tissues not damaged.
- Increases the ability to learn, understand, memorize and retain knowledge.
- Speeds up the reflexes. That is, it improves the function of the brain.
- Improves psychological health.
- Increases the ability to recover from stress in a shorter time than usual.
- Improves the function of the senses and perception in general.
- Allows the individual to enjoy his/her work more and thus derive more satisfaction from work, which increases economic productivity and the quality of life.
- Has a definite role in the treatment of a whole range of illnesses, including hypertension.
- More and more people are reporting the subjective benefits of meditation. Researchers who have been investigating the objective facts find that they too are attracted to meditation by its amazingly large number of positive attributes.

Meditation and the nervous system

The practice of meditation exerts its main influence on the nervous system in the body and is, therefore, so useful in hypertension as it calms the overexcited sympathetic nervous system, reduces the peripheral resistance and drops the blood pressure.

The central nervous system, composed of the brain and spinal cord, sends messages to the peripheral nervous system which is arbitrarily divided into the so-called 'voluntary sensory-motor system and the 'involuntary' autonomic system. The sensory-motor system regulates sensation and willed regulation of muscle, for example, in gross movements such as walking, and in skilled, coordinated, finer movements such as writing. Yoga allows us to become more aware of this

The Brain

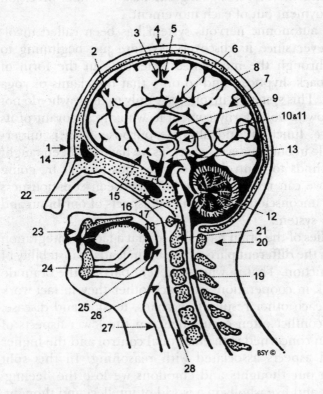

1. Bhrumadhya (eyebrow centre)
2. Frontal lobe (speech, intelligence)
3. Motor cortex (movement)
4. Sahasrara chakra
5. Sensory cortex (sensation)
6. Limbic system (emotion)
7. Occipital lobe (visual)
8. Corpus callosum
9. Thalamus
10. Pineal gland
11. Ajna chakra
12. Cerebellum
13. Hypothalamus
14. Frontal sinus
15. Pituitary gland
16. Sphenoidal sinus
17. Pons
18. Medulla oblongata
19. Spinal cord
20. Atlas vertebra
21. Axis vertebra
22. Nasal cavity
23. Upper lip
24. Tongue
25. Pharynx
26. Larynx and Epiglottis
27. Trachea (to lungs)
28. Oesophagus (to stomach)

system and, therefore, to gain greater control, finer precision and enjoyment out of each movement.

The autonomic nervous system has been called involuntary ever since its discovery. We are just beginning to prove through the medium of science – in the form of biofeedback, hypnosis and so on – that the claims of yoga are true. This system is involuntary only to those who do not know how to voluntarily control it, who are ignorant of its existence, function, and ultimate purpose. This is understandable in our modern society, as we have not been taught the methods to control it. Yoga teaches us that by going inward we can rediscover the links between consciousness and the unconscious, and dormant aspects of our brain and nervous system.

Studies of the brain have shown that a lack of integration between the different parts of the brain leads to instability of body function. That is, when different parts of the brain do not work in cooperation with each other they in fact work against each other resulting in chaos, tension and disease. Such a conflict often occurs between the lower aspects of the brain concerned with emotional control and the higher cerebral aspects associated with reasoning. In this split between our thoughts and emotions we lose the 'feeling' capacity and live wholly in a world of intellect and thought.

The split between thinking and feeling is the precursor of hypertension and all psychosomatic and mental illness. If we think but cannot feel then we do things which we think are good for ourselves but which in reality do our bodies more harm than good. We have lost our sensitivity to our bodies so it becomes hard to know exactly what is healthy and what is destructive. It is only when we relearn through meditation to feel, that our intuition and sensitivity become prominent and take their rightful place. These aspects guide us to do what is right in terms of our own needs; our own evolution. They help us to know ourselves.

If we disregard our feelings then our lives take on destructive patterns. We eat too much, too quickly, or smoke excessively, pollute the atmosphere and in general make life miserable for ourselves. We suffer and do not know why. The reason is that the various parts of our brain are not wired for optimum health and this limits our understanding, reasoning and intuitive powers. We do not know why we become prone to hypertension or how. The fact is that we are responsible for our hypertension and we each have to discover the reasons for ourselves through meditation.

The autonomic nervous system

The autonomic nervous system is linked to the hypothalamus in the brain, which is in turn controlled by the limbic system in the mid brain, the centre concerned with emotions and feelings. The hypothalamus feeds its information into the endocrine glands and the autonomic nervous system, and is the focus point for the union of these two systems. Meditation directly affects the mind/brain complex, calms the hypothalamus and calms the emotions, thereby shutting off excess sympathetic stimulation and hypertension.

The autonomic nervous system can adjust the internal environment according to external and internal needs. It is equipped with two complementary systems. One is the sympathetic nervous system and the other is the parasympathetic. The two subdivisions govern events in the vegetative, or automatic systems, which are normally below the level of consciousness. These branches, the sympathetic and parasympathetic, are mutually antagonistic so that when one is working the other is not. Seen from a different perspective, when one system is active the other is passive. For example, the parasympathetic system causes emptying of the larger bowel and the sympathetic causes retention of the faeces. It is through manipulation of the sympathetic system that one can consciously control the blood pressure. It is thought that the parasympathetic system does not play such a large part in regulation of blood pressure, which is raised by activating the sympathetic nervous system and lowered by turning it off.

The Autonomic Nervous System

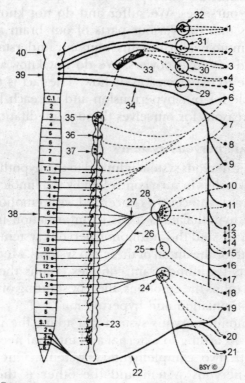

1. Eye	21. Sex organs
2. Lacrimal gland	22. Pelvic nerve
3. Submaxillary gland	23. Sympathetic chain
4. Sublingual gland	24. Inferior mesenteric ganglion
5. Parotid gland	25. Superior mesenteric glanglion
6. Heart	26. Small splanchnic nerve
7. Larynx, trachea, bronchi	27. Greater splanchnic nerve
8. Lung	28. Celiac ganglion
9. Stomach	29. Otic ganglion
10. Small intestine	30. Submaxillary ganglion
11. Abdominal blood vessels	31. Sphenopalatine ganglion
12. Liver	32. Ciliary ganglion
13. Gallbladder	33. Carotid artery and plexus
14. Bile ducts	34. Vagus nerve
15. Pancreas	35. Superior cervical ganglion
16. Adrenal medulla	36. Middle cervical ganglion
17. Kidney	37. Inferior cervical ganglion
18. Colon	38. Spinal cord
19. Rectum	39. Medulla
20. Bladder	40. Midbrain

The following is a list of the functions of the autonomic nervous system:

Parasympathetic component: This system is concerned with relaxation of the body.

- Constricts the pupils
- Secretes tears and saliva
- Constricts the coronary (heart) blood vessels and the bronchi (tubes in the lungs).
- Activates gastric glands in the process of digestion.
- Empties the gallbladder, urinary bladder, stomach, small intestine and large intestine.

Sympathetic component: This system is designed to help the body cope with emergencies and stressful situations.

- Dilates the pupils, allows more light to come in.
- Secretes sweat (anxiety, heat, stressful situations).
- Contracts hair follicles (as in fright).
- Constricts blood vessels to the skin and to the digestive tract directing blood to the more important parts of the body.
- Vasodilates heart and skeletal muscle vessels (preparing the body to fight or flight).
- Increases heart rate pumping more blood and oxygen to the tissues which require more energy.
- Relaxes the bronchial tissue and muscles and dilates bronchi, allowing more oxygen to enter the blood.
- Relaxes the stomach wall, small intestine and colon so that food and faeces can be stored.
- Stores urine in the bladder.
- Mobilizes glucose (sugar) from the liver for extra energy.
- Secretes adrenaline from the adrenal glands.
- Stress raises the blood pressure by constricting the majority of the body's arterioles so that more oxygenated blood can be shunted to the heart, brain and skeletal muscles to react in the best possible way to the environment. It is as though a switch in the brain has been automatically turned in the direction of the sympathetic system, without our control. Yoga enables

117

us to gain control of these brain switches. This is a learned skill which, within the process of evolution, will eventually become second nature to future generations.

Through meditation the mind becomes calmer and clarity of perception increases. Many mental switches come into the field of awareness and we learn to manipulate these. After some time we can lower our blood pressure, aid in digestion, control sweating, heart rate, body temperature, sphincters, hormonal secretions, and many other functions.

Meditation relaxes the mind so that when stressful situations arise you can maintain balance of the autonomic nervous system. This gives you the best view of stress and allows you to cope in the most relaxed possible way. The first step in governing the nervous system is to control the autonomic nervous system, and the means to achieve this is through the practice of meditation.

Meditation

Experiments have shown that the practice of meditation has the following effects:

Metabolic or cell activity is reduced. Meditation decreases oxygen and carbon dioxide utilization in the body, as well as the need for oxygen. A level that is 50 to 75 percent below the scientifically determined minimum for body oxygen requirement can be reached (Anand et.al. 1961 and 1970). This was thought to be impossible without endangering life until masters of yoga showed the opposite to be true.

Wallace and Benson found that in sleep the level of oxygen decreased by approximately 10 percent of the daytime level, while during meditation it decreased by 20 percent, indicating that meditation gives the body greater rest.[32] At the same time carbon dioxide levels decreased by the same amount, indicating that the drop in oxygen did not starve the cells of the body. This shows that meditation is more efficient than sleep in conserving energy.

The brain waves of meditators have been shown through a multitude of experiments to indicate deep relaxation.

118

Increased levels of high amplitude alpha waves, even with the eyes open, have been observed. The average person usually has beta waves predominating, and cannot switch these waves off and on at will. His mind is 'stuck' in an extrovert, tense state. Meditation loosens the mind.

J.P. Banquet found four stages in japa (mantra repetition) meditation.[33] These were:

Stage 1: increased amplitude of alpha waves which moved from the back of the head to the front, indicating relaxation of the worry mechanism in the frontal part of the brain.

Stage 2: theta frequencies different from those of sleep replaced alpha and moved from the frontal part of the brain (intellectual) to the back (occipital or visual) part of the brain. This indicates that the meditator was alert even though he was inside the subconscious mind, responsible for dreams and so on. Theta frequencies occurring in the back of the brain may indicate the time when visions and other psychic phenomena occur in meditation.

Stage 3: rhythmic, synchronous beta waves were present over the whole brain. This seems to indicate that even though the meditator was introvert he was alert and concentrated. The synchronization of brain waves may indicate that all the components of the brain are unifying and reintegrating, removing chaotic, disordered conditioning and making conscious our unconscious potential. There is a subjective sensation of spontaneous creativity and joy that leaves no room for hypertension.

Stage 4: is the emergence into normal waking consciousness through the levels of theta and alpha waves.

The lungs take in less volume of oxygen and the breathing rate is decreased from a normal of 12 to 16 breaths per minute to 4 to 8 per minute during meditation.[34] Other researchers reported that during meditation breathing can drop to as low as one breath per minute or less.

At the same time the resistance to air-entry is reduced by 20 percent which means that air can enter the lungs more easily.[35] This will be of benefit to asthmatics who have much

119

greater air-entry resistance. It is unique to meditation and does not occur in rest.

The heart pumps out less blood as the metabolism is decreased and the body tissues need less oxygen. The tissues have a chance to rest and rebalance, and tissue metabolism can be concentrated on healing. Thomas Routt has reported that the heart rate slows down by about ten beats per minute.[36]

The galvanic skin resistance (GSR) measures the electrical resistance in the skin and the greater the degree of relaxation the greater is the GSR reading. Wallace and Benson found that in meditation the GSR increases by 500 percent, while in sleep it usually only increases by 250 percent.[37]

Lactate, a stress-related chemical, is reduced by meditation. More stress requires more oxygen utilization. Tissue requirement increases until eventually there is not enough oxygen to meet needs. This means that the tissues switch to another energy supply and function less efficiently. They tire faster. Part of this stress mechanism is related to the constriction of the arterioles by the sympathetic nervous system, which prevents the required amount of blood from picking up waste lactate and bringing enough oxygen.

The rate of formation of blood lactate was shown to decrease in the Wallace and Benson study. Its removal from the body during meditation is four times greater than when lying down and resting, and three times faster than its removal in sleep.[38] Relaxation of arterioles washes out the wastes and has beneficial effects on high blood pressure.

Meditation appears to be a unique state which allows greater rest and recuperation from the effects of stress than normal rest or sleep. Wallace and Benson comment:

"There is reason to believe that the changing environment's incessant stimulations to the sympathetic nervous system are largely responsible for the high incidence of hypertension and similar serious diseases that are prevalent in our society.

In these circumstances the hypometabolic state, representing quiescence rather than hyperactivation of the

120

sympathetic nervous system, may indicate a guide post to better health. It should be well worthwhile to investigate the possibilities for clinical application of this state of wakeful rest and relaxation."[39]

Meditators report increased health and wellbeing on both the physical and mental levels of existence, especially decreased numbers of colds, allergies and headaches. Many people are reporting that their blood pressure is no longer a problem since they started to meditate and practise yoga.

Kiely and Gellhorn have found that increased sympathetic stimulation leads to hypertension through increased lability of the autonomic nervous system.[40] K.K. Datey, et al. have shown that through the use of relaxation techniques such as shavasana (closely allied to meditative techniques), high blood pressure was efficiently managed and the drug requirements of successful individuals brought down to as much as 25 percent of the original dose. The blood pressure was brought down by 20 percent to a normal level.[41]

Benson and Wallace have shown in their research that meditators tend to have lower blood pressures.[42] The average of 106/52 mm Hg they found correlates well with the data obtained at the International Yoga Fellowship Movement Research Coordinating Centre, Munger. The usual average in society is 120/80 mm Hg. They then used meditation on their hypertensive patients and found that prior to meditation their pressures were 150 (plus or minus 17)/94 (plus or minus 9) mm Hg. After starting meditation their pressure fell to 141 (plus or minus 11) (88 plus or minus 7) mm Hg, a healthy level, independent of whether the subjects were taking their medication of not.[43] This is a statistically significant decrease of blood pressure and is also significant in that the post meditation diastolic level is below the level arbitrarily designated as hypertensive, 90 mm Hg.

An experiment by one of the associates of the IYFM Research Coordinating Centre in Munger, Dr Shreenivas MD, Director of the Yoga Research Institute, Patna, India (affiliated with Bihar School of Yoga) has also shown that the yogic use of mind is a better way than drugs to reduce blood pressure.

In 150 cases, all males, age group fifteen to forty years, selected at random, he found that the blood pressures were normal, ranging between 100–150/50–80 mm Hg. The average was 120–130/60–70 mm Hg

The subjects were asked to lie down and rest. The blood pressures were again recorded at intervals of ten to thirty minutes until they became established, and this level was taken as the resting blood pressure.

The subjects were then given a tranquilizer 5mg sedative-hypnotic Diazepam) and after waiting for thirty minutes the pressures were recorded. After this, all the men went home to their normal activities and diet. They reported forty-eight hours later for a recheck of their blood pressure.

This time the subjects performed the yogic posture shavasana and did yoga nidra, following the technique of Swami Satyananda Saraswati of the Bihar School of Yoga. These results were obtained:

1. Diazepam had very little effect on blood pressure
2. Yoga nidra brought the blood pressure down by 10–20/ 0–10 mm Hg lower than resting blood pressure.

Dr Shreenivas concluded that yoga nidra is a safe, sound and effective meditation technique for lowering blood pressure. It is described in the practice section of this book.

More experimental evidence is required to differentiate the genuine effects of yoga and meditation from spontaneous cures through drugs and placebo effects of new techniques. It should be emphasized that meditation is not a panacea for all disease, it is not a miracle cure, nor is it a substitute for medication in all psychosomatic illnesses. Rather, it is a way to help speed up nature's processes that lead us back to good health and balance. It is an effective technique that can be utilized to great advantage by all healing communities for speedier and more effective control of hypertension.

Holistic Healing

The word health is derived from the old English word for 'whole', 'holy' or 'complete'. Healing is therefore a means of making ourselves whole, complete and fulfilled human beings. As such it is an ongoing process, for it implies ever-changing patterns of growth and learning. We only attain true health, totality, wholeness when we finally 'grow up' and attain maturity, wisdom and the ability to accept life with all its ups and downs. When we view life from this point to equanimity and detachment (*vairagya*) we are free from the effects of tension and stress that cause hypertension.

To truly grow and come to know ourselves we have to utilize the methods which suit our individual personality and needs. We should not be confined to one system or one method due to an inflexibility of mind. There is no one 'right' system. Whatever works, can be used to eradicate disease. Yoga is open to all systems. Any healing system, whether allopathy, acupuncture or naturopathy, has its place on the tree of healing.

The healing system dominant in the world today is allopathy, the science of curing disease by antagonizing it with drugs, surgery, and so on. When we read the word as *all-opathy* we see it in a different light and it seems to suggest a complete system of healing that incorporates into itself every other system.

123

Traditional science shines its light of research on only a small area of limited knowledge. An experienced scientist would concede that there are realms of understanding which we have only just started to tap and others of which we are completely ignorant. Every system has something to be investigated or to offer, even if it has been derived from sources which are perhaps beyond our experience, but valid nonetheless. Every system must be evaluated for its constructive and creative side so as to eliminate the negative aspects and to incorporate useful, practical ideas into a more complete system. In this way everyone, doctor and patient, healer and healed, would gain the optimum benefits.

Yoga means union, the union of all things in harmony and balance, each in its right place. Then there is no bad or good, no better or worse. We can use whatever healing method we like, when we like and when we need. There are no restrictions or confusions, no stresses or tensions within the healing profession. The root causes of hypertension are eliminated not just at the individual level but also at the global level.

Yoga has as its main advantage that it is a self-healing philosophy. Once you have learned the techniques from an expert you can practise on your own. Your teacher is only a guide, a signpost on the way, to point out your mistakes and faults and to guide you in the best possible direction for the best possible health. You do all the work and thereby gain satisfaction for yourself as well as something no one can ever take away from you, good health, inner security and happiness. Other systems are therefore useful adjuncts to yoga in the short term. They help to reduce the blood pressure during the acute crisis, when you first discover that you have high blood pressure. However, there is no healing method outside yoga that can keep the blood pressure down over a long period of time because only yoga gives us the means to remove the root cause, reorder the brain, rebalance the endocrine system, calm the mind, pacify the emotions, regenerate the pranas.

124

While we are practising the art and the science of yoga, we are treading on a path of knowledge that leads to areas of beauty and peace beyond our expectations. When you are practising the techniques in this book you may also feel like experimenting with other forms of healing.

Acupuncture

One system which is gaining in popularity is that of acupuncture. It is a healing system that has many things in common with yoga. Prana is termed 'chi' in this Chinese philosophy and the dual aspects of nature are called yin and yang, corresponding to the parasympathetic and sympathetic nervous systems, ida and pingala in yoga. Disease is seen to result from abnormalities in the flow of chi, whether excess or deficient.

When disease appears in the body the chi must be rebalanced. Treatment is given using acupuncture needles, massage, herbs or through moxa, a form of heat application. These instruments are applied to points of the body which lie along meridians, or channels of energy, which run throughout the body. Since these channels are equivalent to yogic nadis, yoga and acupuncture may be seen to be complementary.

Both sciences recognize that disease is a process of imbalance and both seek to rebalance the flow of energies. Both are based on a holistic view of the universe, in which the mind and body are seen to be one organ functioning for the use of the soul on an experiential level. If only one aspect of the whole becomes imbalanced disease may result.

Acupuncture sees high blood pressure as caused by excessive heat in the body, emphasizes the removal of this heat, and therefore agrees with the yogic view which states that it is the excessive action of *pingala* (the sun nadi concerned with heating the body) that causes hypertension. Fire, which produces heat, can either be extinguished with water or reduced in intensity by removing some of the wood element which acts as fuel. Using needles or the other tools

125

of acupuncture, the wood element is reduced or the water element is increased. Alternatively the points of the body that correspond to the fire element are stimulated to remove any and all blockages. In the right hands, acupuncture appears to be an effective method.

Physical therapies

This group of therapies includes osteopathy, chiropractic, bioenergetics, biofeedback, Feldenkrais, rolfing and other later developments on the same theme to bring the individual to awareness of his body and its posture, tensions, spasms, distortions, and so on. Many have their base in yoga, or in the universal truth on which yoga is based. Perhaps the most popular of these systems is based on manipulation of the spinal column and the various joints of the body as a means of curing disease.

The correlation between chiropractic and yoga is obvious. Both recognize that a healthy and straight spine is conducive to better health. By freeing the energies of the spine the organs are better controlled by the higher centres of the brain. They are, therefore, better balanced in relation to the other organs of the body and their own internal function to work together.

As in acupuncture, chiropractic and osteopathy deal with energy systems and are the result of experience and insight into the human organism. The results gained from the correct use of these systems have warranted government acceptance and control. Thus chiropractic can be of help to those people seeking to enhance their health through systems other than allopathy, where results in cases of hypertensive disease have not been acceptable to the patient himself, for whom the question of cure is of vital significance. Many people are adopting this method as a means to lower their blood pressure.

Yogasanas are closely related to the osteopathic techniques. They are both based on the structural aspects of the human body and their replacement and manipulation into positions of better function. Asanas have the added advantage of incorporating relaxation and mental concentration, and are a means for the person with high blood pressure to improve his own body. In this way one can gain a great deal of satisfaction and knowledge of the workings of the body. On the other hand, chiropractic depends on expert manipulation of the body from an external source. It is limited to professional practice.

The best means of incorporating yoga and osteopathic treatment is for the chiropractor to utilize his techniques as a means of alleviating acute suffering or for giving the necessary push so that the body can immediately resume a position of better functioning. He should then recommend the use of yogic asana as a method of maintaining this position and preventing problems from recurring. This combination offers fast and sustained relief from suffering and discomfort.

Experimental research into the application of chiropractic has been carried out by workers such as Bandeen, who showed that manipulation of the spine at the level of the eighth to ninth thoracic vertebrae in unselected cases led to a drop in systolic pressure by 10 mm Hg and a drop in diastolic of 5 mm Hg.[44]

Northup demonstrated a more sustained decrease in a small number of cases.[45] Out of 100 cases the average reduction of pressure immediately following the treatment was 33/9 mm Hg.

Norris studied both hypo- and hypertension.[46] He found that hypotensive patients tended to increase their blood pressure while hypertensive patients tended to decrease it. Both improved in the direction of normal which indicates a rebalance of the autonomic nervous system through better alignment of the spinal column. Norris experimented using two groups. One was given manipulation and represented the experimental group. The other group was a control and was told to rest for two hours before their blood pressures were taken. When a comparison was made, the results showed that only 26 percent in the control group lowered their pressures whereas 40 percent of the experimental group gained positive benefits from manipulation. This indicates that the benefits of spinal manipulation are significantly greater than those of simply resting.

Ayurveda

In acupuncture we saw the indigenous Chinese system and its relationship to yoga, while in the physical therapies we saw the techniques developed in Europe and America in attempts to topple the scourge of tension and stress, the foundations of hypertension. The links between these systems and yoga exist because they are based on natural and physiological principles, but are viewed according to the cultural and intellectual climate within which they developed.

The indigenous Indian system of healing is called ayurveda. Because the heritage of yoga was guarded in India over the last five millennia of so, the science of ayurveda grew in contact with yoga and many of the other highly sophisticated philosophies that grew out of the Indian subcontinent, such as vedanta.

The most modern and best known of the ayurvedic texts is the *Charaka Samhita* and the *Susruta*. In these texts all aspects of healing are covered, and are viewed from a natural and holistic perspective. Perhaps the most important concept in ayurveda is that of the *doshas*, the three interconnecting aspects of nature said to be at work in every particle of the human body in different quantities and qualities depending on the part and its function. These three doshas are vata, pitta and kapha.

The word *vata* literally means 'wind'. The *Charaka Samhita* states:"Vata is the source of both structure and function. It is that which is represented by the five forms: prana, udana, samana, vyana and apana. It is the initiator of the upward and downward flow (of all internal processes such as circulation, metabolism, breath, etc.); the controller of the senses; the companion of the sensations; the organizer for the elements of the body; the principle of synthesis; the storage battery of speech; the cause of feelings and perception; the origin of excitement and stimulation. It fans the gastric fire, dries outs harmful phlegm and expels excrement. It is the purifier of the course and fine channels of the body; the creator of foetal form; the principle of life preservation. All theses are normal functions of vata in our body". (Char. Sam.,1–12:8)

Disturbances in vata lead to illnesses such as hypertension and other metabolic and circulatory diseases, emotional or depressive states and everything related to tension, relaxation, expansion, contraction and so on.

The word *pitta* is literally translated as 'bile', which implies the temperament. It is said to be derived from the word *tap*, 'to heat'.

Charaka states: "The results are digestion or indigestion, power of perception and its loss, normal or abnormal body temperatures, healthy or unhealthy looks, fear or courage, joy or anger, clarity or confusion, and other such contrasting pairs." (Char. Sam.,1–12:11)

Diseases resulting from this are: inflammation, fever, pus, bad odour, itching and pain.

The word *kapha* is literally translated as *ka* which means 'water' and *pha* which can be translated as 'the process of biological evolution'. Thus it is 'life-fluid', and has also been called 'phlegm'.

The *Charaka* states that: "Kapha is the nectar. It is fertile water for the play of life; it is living fluid, the protoplasm that sustains all processes; it is the scaffold of life. It binds all the limbs together and produces all the connecting, nourishing, developing and fortifying functions. It promotes the wellbeing of the body by its lubricating process. Thus it supplies the water for the roots of life. In its physiological aspects kapha is the power and perseverance of man, which however, immediately becomes a disturbing impurity when his balance is disturbed." (Char. Sam.,1–12:12)

In disease it manifests as cold, swelling due to fluid, constipation, diabetes and tumours. It is said that there is no pain unless vata is present, no inflammatory process without pitta, and no swellings can occur without kapha.

Ayurveda offers a sophisticated view of the processes of life going on within the body in both its healthy and diseased aspects. A view of health is something that modern allopathy has not achieved. A cure of hypertension is desired but the direction to the cure is missing. We are not exactly sure what 'health' is. Thus allopathy can only gain by investigating and incorporating traditions such as yoga, ayurveda and acupuncture into its fold, updating and making a practical, ideal philosophy for modern man and his hypertension.

Other systems

There are many, many more available health-gaining systems. All have their point of view and deserve a hearing. Homeopathy, for example, is a very subtle but exacting science which has the respect of many doctors, royalty, and indeed most thinking people. Its three basic principles are:
- Like cures like
- The magic of the minimum dose
- Treat the patient and not the disease

It opens up many avenues for the healer to use in his treatment of hypertension.

Another popular method of treatment is naturopathy. This is the science of curing disease through 'natural' methods such as fasting, diet and rest. The natural healers view disease as being caused by toxins and waste matter clogging up the various channels and functions of the body; wrong diet; overeating; use of intoxicants such as tobacco, alcohol, meat, devitaminized foods, synthetic foods and the wrong food combinations, and so on.

The following points comprise naturopathic treatment:
- Diet is regulated. All stimulating drinks and foods are removed from the diet and a similar regimen is followed to the one recommended in this book. However, even in

naturopathy sprouted grains and beans form a major part of the diet, as do raw foods. Fruit fasts and light water fasts are used in conjunction with breathing exercises and sunbathes, and massage is used to help in removal of body toxins.

- Soybeans which contain lecithin, are reputed to be very beneficial for high blood pressure, breaking down cholesterol deposits.
- Herbs such as garlic, hawthorn and valerian are used in high doses. All members of the onion family, consisting of leeks, shallots, chives, garlic, the common onion (brown or white), are of benefit in high blood pressure. They are said to break down cholesterol deposits on the internal surface of the heart and blood vessels. Other herbs used in treatment are: wild cherry bark, rue, broom, boneset, scullcap, red pepper, hyssop and peppermint. They contain chemicals which can soothe the nervous system, cleanse the blood, and heat the circulatory system.
- Red clover tea purifies the blood and is a useful adjunct to the above herbs.
- High herbal enemas clean the colon. This is similar to the hatha yoga cleansing techniques of shankha-prakshalana and basti (shatkarmas).
- Rest in maximum doses is recommended. People are also advised to stop worrying about work and personal problems. However, there in no system in naturopathy to scientifically augment this process. The yogic meditative techniques are an obvious supplement to this deficiency in naturopathy as yoga is itself a natural healing system using natural living as an aid to specific techniques.

The meshwork

All the systems mentioned have many benefits, but they lack one thing. They do not teach us how to dive deep within ourselves and find the cause of our suffering and hyper-tension. Instead they make us dependent on external mediums so that extroversion and imbalance is propagated.

131

For a time we may feel the benefit of other forms of therapy, but eventually we must come back to the realization that only yoga can give us balance and restore harmony. Therefore, yoga should be used as a central core to the removal of hypertension on a long-term basis. All the other methods, whether you choose acupuncture or whatever, are only adjuncts to smooth out and make the process of healing easier. They are short-term methods that the healer may use to finely tune the inner workings, while the major work is done through yoga.

Yoga is a jewel in the desert of hypertension. The many facets of this diamond are reflected in different healing systems, none of which has succeeded in rooting out the cause of hypertension. Those beneficial parts of the systems mentioned are the same as the methods used in yoga, but in the yogic scheme these are all blended into a whole and synthesized to form a multifaceted jewel which shines with its own inner light. Each part of the whole reflects every other part in the light of understanding and awareness.

Practices

Complete Training Program

The following yoga training course for management of high blood pressure must be learned and practised under personal guidance from an expert. The best place is at one of the yoga schools or ashrams affiliated with the Bihar School of Yoga, Munger, where trained sannyasin teachers are available. A list of affiliated institutions can be sent to you on written request from Bihar School of Yoga.

The practices listed here are for reference and guidance only, and we strongly emphasize that you should not practise without expert tuition and supervision. You are also advised to maintain regular contact with your physician in order to gain the best result from this program. If possible, your doctor and yoga teacher should work together so that drug dosages and your condition may be correctly monitored.

Many people who follow the guidance in this book will have already been treated by a qualified medical practitioner and will be taking medication for hypertension. It is necessary to continue this and have your blood pressure checked, and dosage adjusted, at regular intervals:

- Each three days for the first two weeks
- Each week for the next two months
- Then each fortnight for the next two months
- Monthly thereafter until a stable level is reached.

In this way the drugs will be discontinued smoothly and without negative side-effects. When medication has been

135

stopped, daily practice of your yogic sadhana will ensure that your blood pressure remains normal and that you do not need to recommence the drugs.

One of the most important points that we can remember while learning yoga is that the actual time of practice, sadhana, exerts a profound influence on the nervous system, endocrine glands and mind. The effect of sadhana carries over into the rest of the day. If we practise sadhana twice a day the effects are enhanced.

A good suggestion, which cannot be repeated too often, is to practise asana in the morning and before dinner at night for even 5 or 10 minutes, if half an hour or more is not possible. Asana stretch the muscles like a good massage, and a little vajrasana after food aids digestion. These practices also soothe the nervous system and, therefore, the mind. Pranayamas, performed in the morning and before sleep, transform day and night and improve the quality of both our activity and our rest.

The other thing to remember is that we are doing sadhana to transform the quality of our life and experience. The techniques are not the end, only the means, and once we have learnt them they become very much second nature, so that we naturally resort to stretching or gentle breathing the moment our trained awareness picks up some tension. After quite some time of practice we do not even have to think to use these techniques as, through constant practise and repetition, they have become so much a part of our nature that there is no other way we could respond to life, except in an aware and relaxed manner.

Practise simple stretching, body and breath awareness or ajapa japa at any time you remember to do so. Use your watch, for example, as a trigger to remind yourself to practise.

Practice programs

Probably the best and most effective program for people suffering from high blood pressure is pawanmuktasana part 1, nadi shodhana part 2, bhramari pranayama, ajapa japa and yoga nidra. This is especially useful in the more severe forms of hypertension and when there are complications such as heart disease and so on. Occasionally, even pawanmuktasana has to be modified by removing dynamic spinal twist and crow walking exercises due to the effort and strain imposed.

The point to be emphasized time and again is that whatever practice you decide upon, there must be no strain of any kind. Remember the dictum, 'SLOW, RELAXED, AWARE' and you will be sure to benefit. If asanas are performed rapidly, in a tense and emotional frame of mind, benefits are minimal.

Practising asana and pranayama twice a day, especially pranayama and ajapa japa before sleep, will double or triple the benefits of these practices. Asana can be practised before meals in the evening.

Once a basic sadhana is mastered, more practices can be gradually added after a period of a few months or so, again, under expert medical and yogic guidance. Practices such as ajapa japa are a must for uprooting the deeper subconscious disturbances precipitating hypertension. The application of body and breath awareness, as well as mantra, to everyday life will go a long way towards soothing existing tensions and preventing more from building up. These practices above are often enough to slow the brain and mind, relax the body and change our whole attitude toward life and ourselves. In this way we reorient ourselves towards a more total and yogic lifestyle and experience of life.

Eight week intensive program
The following eight week training program is an example of one used for relatively fit people with uncomplicated, mild to moderate hypertension. It is quite complete and demands time, therefore being better suited to people with a genuine desire to change themselves – people who can move outside the confines of the purely physical disease, and dive into the depths of yoga.

137

If such a program is too demanding, or if any problems, strain or exhaustion arise it must be modified, and this can be achieved quite easily by the following suggestions:

1. Substitute the word month for week in the program and you will advance more slowly but surely.
2. After week 5 practise only one round of surya namaskara performing it very slowly and emphasizing gentle stretching, slow breathing and mantra. Remove ujjayi from the pranayama section and practise it only during ajapa japa. Leave out nada, pawan and shabda sanchalana. All of the above suggestions should be carried out in order to create a smaller, balanced program.
3. In week 8 do not start nadi shodhana part 3 unless part 2 has been fully mastered and can be performed 25 times without any effort, strain or feelings of exhaustion or suffocation. If any strain or disturbance occurs in part 3, discontinue and go back to part 2 for another one to three months before commencing part 3.

Remember, in yoga there is no hurry, and a patient attitude of mind combined with regularity of practice, even if it is only ten or twenty minutes of practice per day, will achieve more than irregular but longer, more difficult practice. Patience breeds discipline, determination, fortitude and confidence, and allows ultimately dramatic changes to unfold easily and naturally in life.

First and second weeks

Asana: Pawanmuktasana series as set out in this book.
Vajrasana for ten minutes after each meal. This should be taken up as a daily habit and is therefore mentioned only once.
Shavasana with breath awareness. It is good to practise shavasana in between the other exercises in order to obtain maximum benefits.
Pranayama: Simple regular breathing with deep inhalation and exhalation in the ratio 1:1 either while lying down (in the beginning) or in sitting posture. Practise

alternate abdominal and chest breathing.

Sheetali 5 rounds.

Sheetkari 5 rounds.

Relaxation: Stages 1 and 2 are to be practised for a least ten minutes before going to bed. This technique is easily adapted for use at home or at work, and should be practised at any time you feel tired or tense.

Meditation: ajapa japa, stage 1.

Third and fourth weeks

Asana: Pawanmuktasana

Shavasana with breath awareness.

Surya namaskara up to position 5.

Shavasana.

Pranayama: Regular breathing (see first week).

Ujjayi 21 rounds.

Bhramari 3–5 rounds.

Sheetali 7 rounds.

Sheetkari 7 rounds.

Relaxation: stages 1–4 before sleeping and at any other suitable time during the day.

Meditation: ajapa japa stages 1 and 2.

Fifth and sixth weeks

Asana: Pawanmuktasana.

Surya namaskara complete 1–3 rounds (3 at the end of the fifth week).

Pranayama: Ujjayi up to 49 rounds.

Nadi shodhana stage 1.

Bhramari 7 rounds.

Sheetali 9 rounds.

Sheetkari 9 rounds.

Meditation: Ajapa japa complete in four stages.

Nada sanchalana.

Pawan sanchalana.

Shabda sanchalana.

Yoga nidra.

139

Seventh week

Asana: Pawanmuktasana.
Shavasana.
Surya namaskara 3 rounds.
Pranayama: Ujjayi 49 times.
If meditation is practised after some time, then this ujjayi should be practised up to 108 times.
Nadi shodhana stages 1 and 2.
Bhramari 9 rounds.
Sheetali 9 rounds.
Sheetkari 9 rounds.
Meditation: Ajapa japa complete – 45 minutes.
Yoga nidra complete – 45 minutes.

Eighth week onwards

Asana: Pawanmuktasana and additional shashankasana.
Padmasana.
Surya namaskara 5 rounds.
Shavasana.
Pranayama: Ujjayi 49–108 rounds.
Nadi shodhana stages 1,2 and 3.
Bhramari 9 rounds.
Sheetali and sheetkari 9 rounds each.
Meditation: Ajapa japa complete – 45 minutes.
Yoga nidra complete – 45 minutes.

After the eighth week

You should continue the eighth week program for at least six months. Have your progress checked regularly by your yoga teacher who can make any necessary alterations and adjustments. Visit your doctor too for blood pressure checks and changes in medication.

Asana

The following practice notes should be thoroughly understood before going any further. Although anybody can practise asanas, they become more efficacious and beneficial when performed after correct preparation.

Place: The place where you practise should be clean, quiet and well-ventilated. There should be no bad odour or dampness. The area should be cleared of obstructing furniture and other objects. A blanket or rug should be placed on the floor. Don't use a spongy mattress and do not practise on the bare floor. Try to use the same place every day to build up an atmosphere of peace.

Clothing: Clothing should be as light as possible so free movement is not impeded. Before commencing your practices remove your spectacles, wrist-watch, and any other ornaments or jewellery.

Time: The bowels and bladder should preferably be empty during the practice and the stomach must definitely be empty. (To ensure this allow three to four hours after taking food.) It is thus best to practise in the early morning before breakfast. This also allows the practitioner to take advantage of brahmamuhurta (between four and six o'clock) which is the time of day most conducive to yoga practices. Although the body is stiffer in the morning, there are fewer distractions and the atmosphere is pure and quite. However, asanas can be practised any time of day except after meals.

Duration: The duration of practice should be regulated according to available time. Don't set your aims high in the beginning; only do as much practice as you can do regularly, every day, without fail. Fifteen minutes practice every day is better than one hour of practice one day, none for three days and again one hour.

Sequence: You should begin your program with asanas, followed by pranayama and then meditation. Of course, if time is limited, you may begin meditation without preliminary practices.

Limitations: Don't practise asana if you are ill with a cold, diarrhoea or something similar. At these times the body is directing its energy to specific areas to fight the illness; let it perform its duties unimpeded.

Slow, controlled movement: In order to bring about harmony and gain the most benefit from asanas, they should be practised with slow, controlled movements coordinated with the breath. Fast movements imply excessive tension and quick, sudden movements use up excessive energy. Asanas aim at conserving energy and developing muscular control, both of which come from slow, mindful practice. During slow movement it is possible to relax the maximum number of muscles that are not directly involved in the particular asana. In each asana breathing instructions have been included to facilitate this coordination and relaxation, and they should be followed as closely as possible. Breathe only through the nose.

Maintenance of final pose: The final position is the most important part of the practice. This period of immobility is the time when profound and beneficial changes are occurring in the body.

Relaxation: Never exert any undue force or strain while doing asanas. Athough most beginners will find their muscles stiff to start with, they will definitely become more supple with regular practice. Relax the muscles in order to stretch them. If your muscles are tense they will resist stretching. Relaxation between asanas is just as important as the asana

142

itself. When one completely relaxes, the organs and muscles return to their normal shape and they are flooded with purified blood to replace that squeezed out during execution of the asanas. During this rest period the circulatory and respiratory systems also return to normal.

Asanas are really relaxation postures. However, shavasana is an important resting pose and should be practised between asanas. It is also a part of many short relaxation techniques and is the ideal sleeping position. This posture gives complete support to the spine and is scientifically approved for ensuring maximum rest during sleep.

Awareness: While learning the asana your attention should be on correct performance. In the final position you can be aware of the breath, mantra, or particular parts of the body that the asana especially influences. Such awareness is most useful in directing the body's natural healing energies.

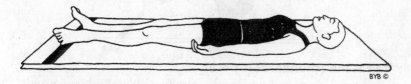

Shavasana (corpse pose)

Lie flat on the back with the arms beside and in a line with the body and with the palms facing upward.

Move the feet slightly apart to a comfortable position.

Close the eyes and relax the whole body.

Do not move any part of the body even if discomfort arises.

Let the breath become rhythmic and natural.

Let the mind become aware of inhalation and exhalation.

Count the number of breaths – 1 in, 1 out; 2 in, 2 out; and so on.

Continue to count for a few minutes; if the mind begins to wander, bring it back to the counting.

Maintain this pose as long as you feel necessary. Your

body will tell you when it is rested. During asana practice a few minutes is usually sufficient. After asana practice rest a little longer.

This pose fully relaxes the psychophysical system. It is ideally practised before sleep, before or during asana and particularly after a dynamic exercise such as surya namaskara.

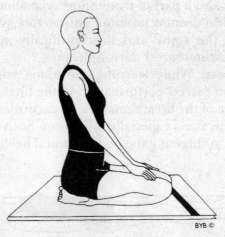

BYB ©

Vajrasana (thunderbolt pose)

Stand on your knees with your feet stretched backwards and your big toes crossed.

Your knees should be together and your heels should be apart.

Lower your buttocks onto the insides of your feet.

Your heels will be at the side of your hips.

Place your hands on your knees with the palms downwards.

Your breath should be normal. Try to feel the movement of the abdominal muscles and direct the awareness to the lower abdomen.

You can sit in this pose at any time of the day when you have a spare moment. It is to be especially utilized for ten to fifteen minutes after a meal, as an aid to the digestive process.

144

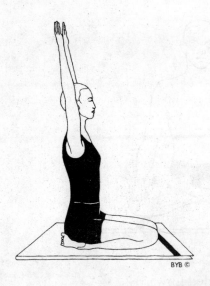

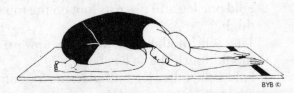

Shashankasana (pose of the moon or hare pose)

Sit in vajrasana, placing the hands on the knees.

While inhaling, raise the arms so that they are above the head.

Exhale while bending the trunk forward, keeping the arms in line with the trunk; at the end of the movement the hands and forehead should rest on the floor.

Retain the breath for a short time in the final position.

Breathe in while returning slowly to the upright position.

Slowly return to the starting position while exhaling.

The breath should be slow and coordinated with the physical movement.

Normal or even, slow, deep breathing may be practised in the prostrated stage if it is maintained for a longer period of time.

145

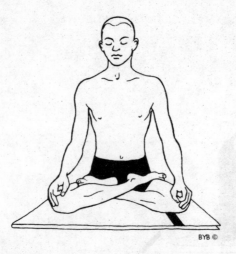

BYB ©

Padmasana (lotus pose)

Sit with your legs extended forward.

Fold one leg and place its foot on the top of the opposite thigh.

The sole of the foot must be upward and the heel should touch the pelvic bone.

Fold your other leg and place its foot on the top of the other thigh.

The spine must be steady and completely upright as though fixed to the ground.

This posture is easier to maintain if a low cushion is placed under the buttocks before assuming the pose.

Precautions: This asana should not be attempted until the practitioner has developed suppleness of the legs through the regular practice of the other asanas mentioned in the practice program, or learned from a teacher.

Practice note: Padmasana can be practised in conjunction with either jnana or chin mudra. Jnana mudra places the hands palms down, while chin mudra places the hands palms up. In both, the index fingers are curled and folded so that they touch either the top or the root of their respective thumbs.

146

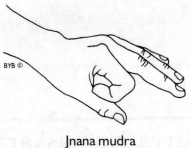

Jnana mudra

If padmasana is too difficult, use ardha padmasana (one leg on top of the opposite thigh, the other leg under the buttocks of the opposite side), sukhasana (easy, cross-legged pose) or some other variation.

Surya Namaskara

Surya namaskara revitalizes the whole body, loosens all the joints, flexes every muscle in the body, and activates the respiratory and circulatory systems. It also balances the flow of prana in the ida and pingala nadis, providing optimum conditions for meditation. The practice consists of five essential aspects.

Physical postures: There are twelve physical postures which correspond to the signs of the zodiac.

Breathing: Each position is associated with either inhalation, retention or exhalation of breath, so that the whole sequence is synchronized with breathing. This breath flow must not be forced or unnatural.

Mantra: Associated with each position is a mantra which is uttered mentally or out loud. A mantra is a combination of sounds, syllables or phrases which have been heard in deepest meditation by saints and sages. They are evocative sounds which, through the power of vibration, have subtle, yet potent and penetrating effects on mind and body.

Awareness: This is as essential in surya namaskara as it is in all yogic practices. Concentration and awareness are used to gain maximum benefit from the practices.

Relaxation: Relaxation is necessary on completion of the practice to allow the body to calm itself and integrate the benefits gained. Shavasana with constant awareness of the breath is the most recommended posture.

Sequence for learning

One should first familiarize oneself with the twelve positions and for at least a week be concerned only with mastering the physical movements. Once you find that you can perform all the movements automatically with little conscious direction, then synchronize the breath. Awareness should then be on both breath and movement. Finally learn the mantras and try to synchronize them with each position.

One complete round

One complete round consists of twenty-four poses. We have given twelve .positions, with the right leg brought forward and the left leg stretched behind in the lunging positions (4 and 9). These same twelve positions are to be repeated, but with the opposite side of the body, the left leg lunging forward and the right leg extended backward.

Tempo and number of rounds

At first surya namaskara should be performed slowly to ensure correct development of the movement and breathing. However, with regular practice your body will flow smoothly through the positions and you will be able to perform them faster. You may then speed up the practice but always ensure that the breath does not become shallow and that the mantras are correctly pronounced.

The number of rounds depends on individual health and time available. In hypertension it is rare to do more than five rounds, especially within the first six months of practice. Most people should perform only one or two rounds very slowly, remaining in the final relaxed pose for a few seconds and breathing normally. Never practise to exhaustion and always perform shavasana at the end of the series for three to five minutes.

If at any stage of this practice you experience any doubts, difficulties or ill-effects, then stop the practice and seek expert guidance.

149

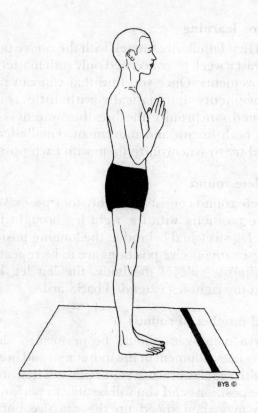

BYB ©

Position 1: **Pranamasana (prayer pose)**
Stand erect with the feet together.
Place the palms together in front of the chest.
Relax the whole body.
Breath: Normal.
Concentration: Anahata chakra.
Mantra: *Om Mitraya Namaha*, salutations to the friend
of all.

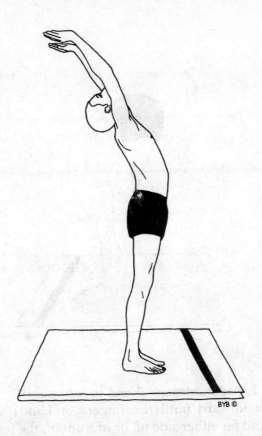

Position 2: Hasta Utthanasana (raised arms pose)

Raise both arms above the head.

Keep the arms separated by one shoulder's width.

Bend the head and upper trunk slightly backwards.

Breath: Inhale while raising the arms.

Concentration: Vishuddhi chakra.

Mantra: *Om Ravaye Namaha*, salutations to the shining one.

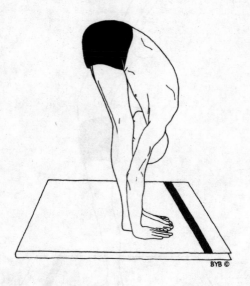

Position 3: Padahastasana (hand to foot pose)
Bend forward until the fingers or hands touch the ground on either side of, or in front of, the feet.
Try to touch the knees with the forehead, but do not strain. Keep the legs straight.
Breath: Exhale as you bend forward. Try to contract the abdomen in the final position.
Concentration: Swadhisthana chakra.
Mantra: *Om Suryaya Namaha*, salutations to the giver of energy.

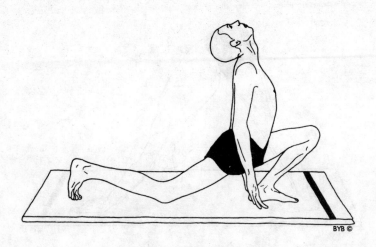

Position 4: Ashwa Sanchalanasana (equestrian pose)
Stretch the right leg back as far as possible.
At the same time bend the left leg, but keep the left foot
in the same position.
The arms should remain straight in the same position.
At the end of the movement the weight of the body
should be supported on the two hands, the left foot, the
right knee and the toes of the right foot.
In the final position the head should be tilted backwards,
the back arched and the gaze directed upwards.
Breath: Inhale whilst you stretch the right leg backwards.
Concentration: Ajna chakra.
Mantra: *Om Bhanave Namaha*, salutations to he who illumines
the infinite universe.

153

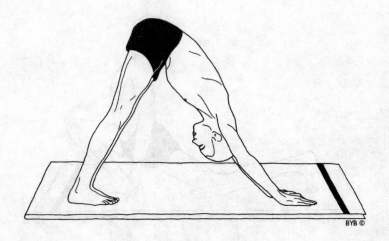

Position 5: Parvatasana (mountain pose)
Straighten the left leg and place the left foot beside the
right foot. Raise the buttocks in the air and lower the
head between the two arms; with legs and arms straight,
and heels in contact with the floor, the body should
form two sides of a triangle.

Breath: Breathe out as you straighten the left leg and then
bend the trunk.

Concentration: Vishuddhi chakra.

Mantra: *Om Khagaya Namaha*, salutations to the one who
moves quickly in the sky.

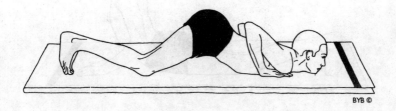

BYB ©

Position 6: Ashtanga Namaskara (salute with eight parts or points)

Lower the body to the ground, so that in the final position of the pose only the toes of both feet, the two knees, the chest, the hands and the chin touch the ground.

The hips and abdomen should be raised slightly off the ground.

Breath: The breath should be held outside. No respiration.

Concentration: Manipura chakra.

Mantra: *Om Pushne Namaha*, salutations to the giver of strength.

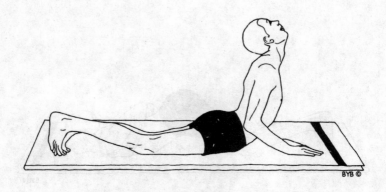

Position 7: Bhujangasana (serpent pose).

Raise the body from the waist by straightening the arms.

Bend the head backwards.

Breath: Inhale while raising the body and arching the back.

Concentration: Swadhisthana chakra.

Mantra: *Om Hiranyagarbhaya Namaha*, salutations to the golden cosmic self.

Position 8: Parvatasana (mountain pose)

From the arched back position assume the mountain pose as described in position 5.

Breath: Exhale as you raise the buttocks in the air.

Concentration: Vishuddhi chakra.

Mantra: *Om Marichaya Namaha*, salutations to the lord of the dawn.

Position 9: Ashwa Sanchalana (equestrian pose)

As for position 4, bend the left leg and bring the left foot forwards so that it lies near the hands.

Simultaneously lower the right knee to the floor.

Breath: Inhale while assuming the pose.

Concentration: Ajna chakra.

Mantra: *Om Adityaya Namaha*, salutations to the son of Aditi.

Position 10: Padahastasana (hand to the foot pose)

This position is a repeat of position 3.

Place the right foot next to the left foot.

Straighten both the legs and try to bring the forehead as close as possible to the knees. Do not strain.

Breath: Exhale while performing the movement.

Concentration: Swadhisthana chakra.

Mantra: *Om Savitre Namaha*, salutations to the benevolent mother.

Position 11: Hasta Utthanasana (raised arms pose)

As for position 2, straighten the whole body and raise the arms above the head.

Bend the head and arms backward slightly.

Breath: Inhale as you straighten the body.

Concentration: Vishuddhi chakra.

Mantra: *Om Arkaya Namaha*, salutations to he who is fit to be praised.

Position 12: Pranamasana (prayer pose)
   This is the final pose and is the same as position 1.
Breath: Exhale as you assume the final pose.
Concentration: Anahata chakra.
Mantra: *Om Bhaskaraya Namaha,* salutations to the one who
   leads to enlightenment.

Pawanmuktasana

This series of exercises is especially designed for those people who are suffering from hypertension. It differs from the usual series, for exercises which place undue stress and strain on the circulatory system have been removed. This series has always been found to be useful for those people who are beginners and whose bodies are too stiff to attempt major asana immediately on commencing yoga.

Though it seems to be nothing more than a series of joint rotations and limbering up exercises, the pawanmuktasana series works directly on the pranic energy systems of the body. It systematically loosens up the joints from the big toe to the head and neck, removing those tensions which hold our bodies stiff and rigid and prevent energy from flowing adequately. At the same time pawanmuktasana acts on the cortex of the brain, systematically enervating the cortex responsible for sensation and motion. We thereby reorder the neuronal circuits, leading to more mental peace, order and equanimity.

Thus pawanmuktasana is the ideal series for the hypertensive person. It not only systematically calms the whole body from head to toe, but it also relaxes the entire blood vessel system. It can be used after a long period in bed to aid convalescence. Practise this series with full awareness, integrating body, breath and mind, and enjoying the extra energy and relaxation you will feel.

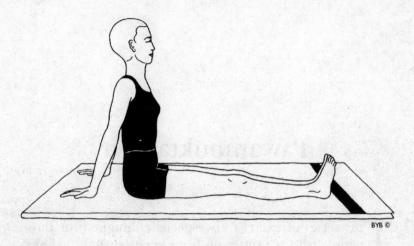

Pararambhik Sthiti (base position)

Sit with your legs extended in front of the body. This is the base position. Place your hands on the floor by the side of the trunk, lean backwards, and take the support of the straight arms.

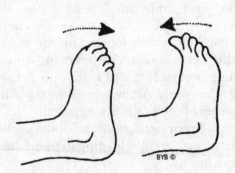

Exercise 1: Padanguli Naman (toe bending)

Become aware of the toes.
Move the toes of both feet slowly backwards and forwards, keeping the feet rigid.
Repeat ten times.

160

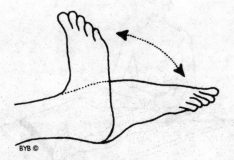

Exercise 2: Goolf Naman (ankle bending)

Remain in the base position.

Move both feet backward and forward as much as possible, bending them from the ankle joints.

Feel the stretch forward over the instep, and the backward pull on your calf muscle.

Repeat ten times.

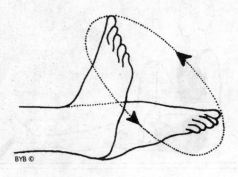

Exercise 3: Goolf Chakra (ankle rotation)

Remain in the base pose.

Separate the legs, keeping them straight.

Keeping the heels in contact with the floor, rotate the right foot clockwise about the ankle, ten times. Then rotate the same foot anticlockwise, ten times.

Repeat the same procedure with the left foot.

Repeat the exercise, but rotating both feet together.

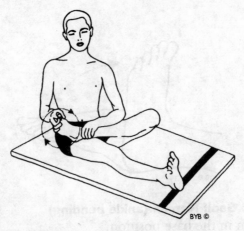

Exercise 4: Goolf Ghoornan (ankle crank)

Assume the base posture.

Place the right ankle on the left thigh.

With the assistance of the left hand, rotate the right foot clockwise ten times, then ten times anticlockwise.

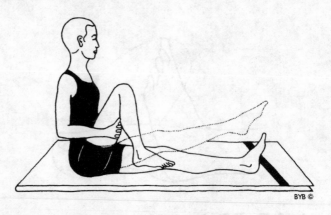

Exercise 5: Janu Naman (knee bending)

Assume the base position.

Bend the right leg at the knee and clasp your hands under the right thigh.

Straighten your right leg without allowing the heel or toe to touch the ground, keeping the hands under the right thigh but allowing the arms to straighten.

Bend the right leg as much as possible at the knee,

162

bringing the heel near the right buttock.

Repeat ten times each leg.

Variation: Assume the base position.

Instead of stretching the right leg, hold the thigh near the trunk and rotate the lower leg in circular motion about the knee.

Do ten times clockwise and ten times anticlockwise.

Repeat the same procedure with the left leg.

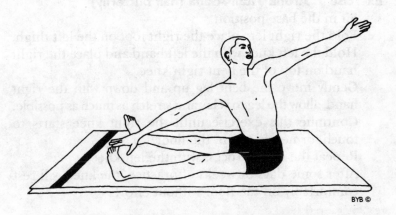

BYB ©

Exercise 6: Gatyatmak Meru Vakrasana (dynamic spinal twist)

Assume the base position.

Separate the legs as much as you comfortably can.

Keeping the arms straight, bring the left hand to the right big toe and stretch the right arm behind the back, keeping both arms in one straight line.

Look backwards, directing the gaze to the right hand.

Turn the trunk in the opposite direction, bring the right hand to the left big toe and stretch your left arm behind you.

This is one round.

Repeat a maximum of five times on each side.

Now practise shavasana for a few minutes.

163

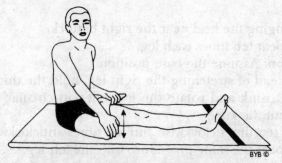

Exercise 7: Ardha Titali Asana (half butterfly)

Sit in the base position.

Fold the right leg, place the right foot on the left thigh.
Hold the left knee with the left hand and place the right
hand on top of the bent right knee.

Gently move the bent leg up and down with the right
hand, allow the leg to relax and stretch as much as possible.
Continue this exercise until the right knee starts to
touch, or nearly touch, the floor.

Repeat the same process with the left knee.

After some days or weeks of practice, the knee will rest
comfortably on the floor without effort.

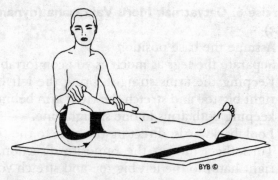

Exercise 8: Shroni Chakra (hip rotation)

Remain in the same position as exercise 7, but hold the
right toes with the left hand.

Rotate the right knee in a circle, ten times clockwise and
then ten times anticlockwise.

Repeat with the left knee.

164

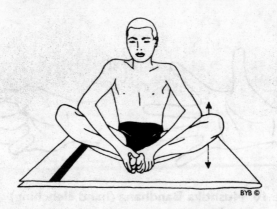

Exercise 9: Poorna Titali Asana (full butterfly)

Sit erect and bring the soles of the feet together.
Try to bring the heels as close to the body as possible.
Interlock the fingers and place them under the feet.
Then gently push the knees to the ground, by using the
elbows.
While pushing the knees downward try to bend the
body forward and touch the ground with the head.

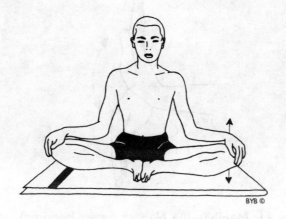

Now place the hands on the knees.
Using the arms, push the knees to the floor, and allow
them to bounce up again.
Repeat twenty times or more.

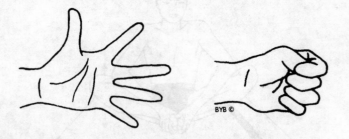

Exercise 10: Mushtika Bandhana (hand clenching)

Assume the base position.

Hold the arms straight in front of the body, so that they are in line with the shoulders.

Stretch and tense the fingers of both hands.

Close the fingers over the thumbs and make a tight fist.

Again stretch and tense the fingers. Repeat this ten times, with full awareness.

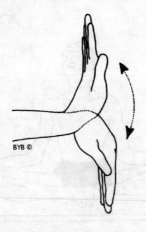

Exercise 11: Manibandha Naman (wrist bending)

Bend the hands at the wrist, as if you are pressing the palms against a wall.

From the upward-pointing of the fingers, bend the hands at the wrist and point the fingers downwards.

Repeat this ten times.

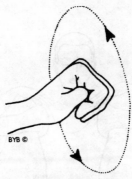

Exercise 12: Manibandha Chakra (wrist joint rotation)

Stay in the same position as exercise 11, but with only the right hand extended.

Clench the right fist and rotate it clockwise ten times about the wrist.

Then rotate the fist anticlockwise ten times. Repeat with the left hand.

Extend both arms in front of the body with fists clenched. Rotate the fists together, ten times clockwise then ten times anticlockwise. Lower the arms and relax before commencing the next exercise.

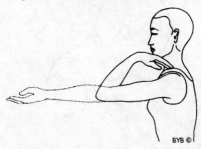

Exercise 13: Kehuni Naman (elbow bending)

Hold both arms outstretched with the palms up.

Bend both arms at the elbows and touch the shoulders with the fingers.

Straighten the arms once again.

Repeat ten times.

Perform the same movement with arms extended sideways, ten times.

167

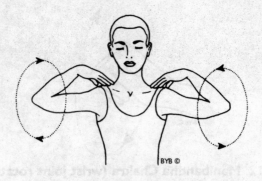

Exercise 14: Skandha Chakra (shoulder socket rotation)

Stay in the same position as previously.

Make a circular movement from the shoulders joints, keeping your fingers in contact with the shoulders.

Try to bring the elbows into contact in front of the chest.

Do this ten times clockwise, ten times anticlockwise.

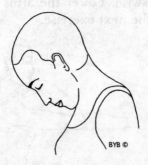

Exercise 15a: Greeva Sanchalana (neck movements)

Place your hands on the floor by your thighs in the sitting position, and keep your legs straight. Slowly move your head backwards and forwards.

Repeat ten times.

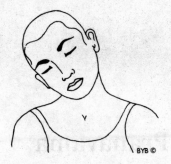

Exercise 15b

Slowly tilt your head to the left and to the right, first while facing directly forward.

Then turn the head slowly from left to right.

Practise each method ten times.

Pranayama

Pranayama, correctly used, is the bridge between body and mind. It should be done gently, with awareness. It should never be forced in the expectation of better results, as this is a block to success. It is better to practise below your maximum capacity at first so that you do not suffer strain.

Pranayama also brings tranquility and restricts interference from the thought process. It stills the disturbances of the mind, freeing us to tune in to the subtle aspects of our being. Pranayama is, therefore, a vital technique for all those who would tread the spiritual path.

The following points should be carefully read and observed before starting pranayama:

- The bladder, stomach and intestines should be empty before doing pranayama. Wait for at least four hours after meals.
- Do pranayama after asana but before meditation practices.
- While doing pranayama the body should be relaxed. Spine, neck and head should be erect and centred.
- During pranayama there should be no strain. Breath retention should not be done for longer than is comfortable. This is most important for the lungs are very delicate organs and any misuse can easily cause them to be injured.
- Practise in a well-ventilated (not windy), clean and pleasant environment.

- When beginning **pranayama** some constipation and a reduction in the quantity of urine may be experienced. In the case of dry motions, stop taking salt and spices. If you have a loose motion, then stop pranayama for a few days and take to a diet of rice and curd (yoghurt).
- Cover the body with a comfortable garment, sheet or blanket so that there are no external disturbances such as insects during the practices.

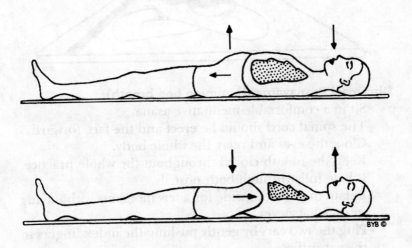

Yogic breathing

Inhale by first expanding the abdomen and then the chest in one slow, smooth motion until the maximum possible amount of air has been drawn into the lungs. Then exhale and allow the air to passively escape from the lungs. This should be accompanied by a feeling of letting go and relaxation. Inhalation is active, exhalation passive.

The whole movement should be smooth (no jerks) from the abdomen to the chest, like a wave.

This procedure should be repeated for all inhalations and exhalations during the entire day.

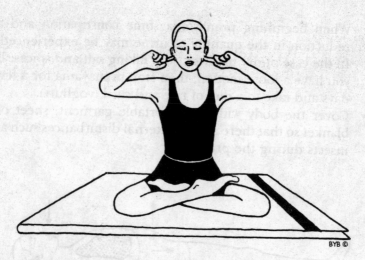

Bhramari Pranayama (humming bee breath)

Sit in a comfortable meditative asana.

The spinal cord should be erect and the face forward.

Close the eyes and relax the whole body.

Keep the mouth closed throughout the whole practice.

Inhale fully through both nostrils.

Retain the breath inside for a few moments without any strain whatsoever.

Plug the two ears by gently pushing the index fingers in the ear orifices.

Keep the mouth closed, separate the teeth and then slowly exhale producing a long continuous humming sound like a bee.

The exhalation should be slow and steady.

Feel the vibrations of the sound in the brain and be conscious only of the sound. This is the end of one round.

Start with five rounds and slowly increase the number.

Do not do this practice in a prone position, for the glottis would be placed under tension.

Do not strain the lungs in any way.

172

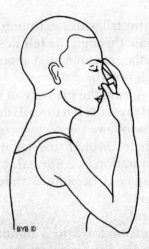

Hand position: Nasagra Mudra (nosetip position)

Hold the fingers of the right hand in front of the face. Rest the index and middle fingers gently on the eyebrow centre. Both fingers should be relaxed.

The thumb is above the right nostril and the ring finger above the left. These two digits control the flow of breath in the nostrils by alternately pressing on one nostril, blocking the flow of breath, and then the other.

The little finger is comfortably folded. When practising for long periods, the elbow may be supported by the left hand although care is needed to prevent chest restriction.

Nadi Shodhana Pranayama (psychic network purification)
Technique 1: Preparatory practice

Sit in any comfortable meditation posture, preferably siddha/siddha yoni asana or padmasana. (Those who cannot sit in a meditation posture may sit against a wall with the legs outstretched or in a chair which has a straight back). Keep the head and spine upright.

Relax the whole body and close the eyes.

Practise yogic breathing for some time.

Adopt nasagra mudra with the right hand and place the left hand on the knee in chin or gyana mudra.

173

Close the right nostril with the thumb.

Inhale and exhale through the left nostril 5 times.

The rate of inhalation/exhalation should be normal.

Be aware of each breath.

After 5 breaths release the pressure of the thumb on the right nostril and press the left nostril with the ring finger, blocking the flow of air.

Inhale and exhale through the right nostril 5 times, keeping the respiration rate normal.

Lower the hand and breathe 5 times through both nostrils together.

This is one round.

Practise 5 rounds or for 3 to 5 minutes, making sure there is no sound as the air passes through the nostrils.

After practising for 15 days go on to technique 2.

Technique 2: Alternate nostril breathing

In this technique the duration of inhalation/exhalation is controlled.

Close the right nostril with the thumb and breathe in through the left nostril.

At the same time count mentally, "1, Om; 2, Om; 3, Om", until the inhalation ends comfortably. This is the basic count.

Breathe deeply with yogic breathing. Do not strain.

Close the left nostril with the ring finger, release the pressure of the thumb on the right nostril and while breathing out through the right nostril, simultaneously count, "1, Om; 2, Om; 3, Om". The time for inhalation and exhalation should be equal.

Next, inhale through the right nostril, keeping the same count in the same manner.

At the end of inhalation close the right nostril, open the left nostril and exhale through the left nostril, counting as before.

This is one round.

Practise 10 rounds.

174

Ratio and timing: After a few days, if there is no difficulty, increase the length of inhalation/exhalation by one count. Continue in this way, increasing the inhalation/exhalation by one count as it becomes easy, until the count of 24:24 is reached.

Do not force the breath in any way and be careful not to speed up the counting during exhalation to compensate for shortage of breath. At the slightest sign of discomfort reduce the count.

After perfecting the above ratio, it may be changed to 1:2. For example, breathe in for a count of 4 and breathe out for a count of 8 or breathe in for a count of 5 and breathe out for a count of 10 and so on. This ratio establishes a calming rhythm for the brain and heart, assisting the treatment of cardiovascular and nervous system disorders specifically, and stress related conditions generally.

When this technique can be performed with complete ease move on to technique 3.

Technique 3: with Antar Kumbhaka (inner retention)

In this technique antar kumbhaka or internal breath retention is introduced.

Close the right nostril and breathe in slowly through the left nostril for a count of 5.

At the end of inhalation, close both nostrils and retain the air in the lungs for a count of 5.

The glottis may be slightly contracted to hold the air within the lungs.

Open the right nostril, breathe in slightly through the right nostril and then slowly breathe out through the same nostril for a count of 5.

This slight inhalation at the end of inner retention helps to bring the respiratory muscles back into action again and relieves the locked condition of the glottis.

The exhalation should be smooth and controlled and of the same length as the inhalation.

175

At the end of exhalation, immediately inhale through the right nostril for a count of 5, keeping the left nostril closed.

Again, retain the breath for a count of 5 with both nostrils closed.

Open the left nostril, breathe in slightly through the left nostril and then breathe out through the same nostril for a count of 5.

This is one round.

Maintain constant awareness of the count and of the breath.

Practise 10 rounds.

Ratio and timing: The maintenance of a strict ratio during inhalation, kumbhaka and exhalation is of the utmost importance. The ratio will change as the ability to hold the breath for longer periods of time progressively develops. After mastering the ratio of 1:1:1, increase the ratio to 1:1:2. For example, inhale for a count of 5, perform internal kumbhaka for a count of 5 and exhale for a count of 10. After some weeks of practice, when this ratio has been mastered, increase the ratio to 1:2:2. Inhale for a count of 5, do internal kumbhaka for a count of 10 and exhale for a count of 10.

After mastering the ratio of 1:2:2, gradually increase the count by adding one unit to the inhalation (e.g. 5 becomes 6), 2 units to the retention and 2 units to the exhalation (making each of them 12). The count of one round will then be 6:12:12. Practise this stage until it is mastered.

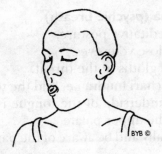

Sheetali Pranayama (cooling breath)

Sit in any meditative pose.

Place the palms on the knees.

Poke out the tongue and fold the sides to form a narrow tube.

Inhale slowly and deeply through the folded tongue.

Retain the breath for a few moments.

After a short time exhale through the nose as slowly as you comfortably can.

Inhale through the folded tongue and repeat.

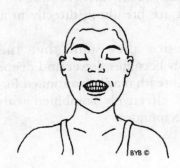

Sheetkari Pranayama (hissing breath)

This is similar to sheetali pranayama and it is done the same way except for the position of the tongue.

The tongue should be folded backwards so that the lower surface touches the upper palate. Clench the teeth together and keep the lips apart.

The inhalation should be through the teeth.

177

Ujjayi Pranayama (psychic breath)

Sit in any meditative posture.

Relax, and close your eyes.

Contract the glottis in the throat.

Perform khechari mudra i.e. fold the tongue backwards so that the underside of the tongue is pressed against the back of the upper palate.

Inhale naturally and be aware of the passage of breath in the throat.

If the glottis is properly contracted you will hear a very soft, gentle, snoring sound like the sound of a distant waterfall, or of a sleeping baby.

Exhale naturally, again with awareness of the breath in the throat and the sound of your breathing.

Do not strain – this sound should be loud enough only for yourself to hear.

Continue in this way – natural, spontaneous breathing with the throat contracted and the tongue in khechari mudra.

Try to feel that you are not breathing through the nose, but that you are breathing directly in and out of the throat.

You will notice after some time that the breath spontaneously becomes slower and deeper.

This psychic breath may be continued for as long as you wish, and is effectively combined with mudras and meditative techniques.

Meditation Practice

Stage 1: Lie in a comfortable position.

Adjust your position if you need to.

Close your eyes and relax yourself completely.

Become aware of your whole body.

Feel that your body is part of the ground.

Feel all the sensations of your body and, if possible, try to create a mental image of your body.

Be aware of any aches or pains.

Direct your awareness to the source of this discomfort and try to be aware of nothing else.

Let this pain be a focus for your awareness.

If your mind starts to wander, let it, but simultaneously try to maintain your awareness of the pain in the body.

Continue for a few minutes.

Then direct your awareness to your right foot.

Be aware of nothing else but your right foot.

After a short time, transfer awareness to your left foot.

You can create a mental picture of the left foot and feel the sensations connected with it. Remain aware.

Transfer your awareness to your right leg and repeat the process.

Repeat with your left leg, the abdomen, chest, right arm, left arm, neck, head and finally the whole body.

This is one round.

Intensify your awareness.

179

Although your awareness may stray onto other subjects, continue to be aware of your body.

Do another round, and be aware.

Move your awareness to different parts of the body.

Try to feel the different parts of the body as you have never felt them before.

In this way continue your practice.

Stage 2: Close your eyes.

Become aware of breathing.

Imagine that you are breathing in and out from the heart. Breathe directly from the heart.

You must count each of your inhalations and exhalations from fifty back to zero.

As you inhale, count fifty.

As you exhale, count forty-nine.

As you inhale again, count forty-eight.

Continue in this way to zero, maintaining awareness of the breathing process and mental counting.

Your breath should be natural.

If you lose count, start again.

Do this for as long as you have time available.

Stage 3: This practice is the same stage 2, but you must imagine that the exhalation and inhalation move in and out to the throat (vishuddhi chakra).

Stage 4: Be aware of the flow of breath through the nostrils, carefully noting all sensations.

As you breath in, count fifty.

As you breathe out, count forty-nine.

Continue in this manner until you reach zero.

You must maintain awareness of the flow of breath through the nostrils and mental counting.

Ajapa japa

Japa is the constant repetition of a mantra. Japa becomes ajapa (spontaneous) when the mantra repeats itself automatically, without any conscious effort. This technique uses the spontaneous mantra of the breath, *Soham*, to calm the mind and to transfer this mental tranquility to the body, effecting healing at the deepest level of being.

During the preliminary practice of ajapa japa, the practitioner should try to feel the prana (healing bioenergy) flowing in the frontal psychic passage that runs between the navel and the throat. Your teacher will help you to locate this passage. Initially you will need to use your imagination, but later this pranic passage will become a reality for you.

Awakening prana in the frontal psychic passage and in the spinal cord rebalances the body, increases energy and purifies the mind so that the whole organism functions at a healthier, more efficient level. Your illness will rapidly be replaced by an experience of joy and vitality.

Stage 1: Sit in a comfortable position.

Close your eyes and relax the whole body.

Hold the spine upright, but without excessive strain. Tell yourself that for the duration of the practice all problems and worries will be discarded; all attention will be on the practice of ajapa japa.

When you are ready, start the practice.

Do ujjayi pranayama and khechari mudra. (Roll the tongue backwards so that the normally lower surface touches the upper palate. Try to bring the tongue back as far as possible without strain.)

Become aware of your breathing process.

As you breathe in, know that you are breathing in.

When breathing out, know you are breathing out.

Be totally attentive to every incoming and outgoing breath; feel the rhythm of the flow.

Carry on in this manner for a few minutes.

Then imagine that the breath is flowing between the navel and the front of the throat.

On inhalation, the breath ascends from the navel to the throat.

On exhalation, the breath descends from the throat to the navel.

181

At first you may find this process difficult to imagine. Don't worry, only try. The important thing is to be completely aware of the breath.

Let the breathing become rhythmical, deep and long, but without force. The more you relax, the more the breath will automatically become slow and deep.

Continue in this manner for at least five minutes. Maintain awareness.

If the mind wanders, which it surely will, don't fight it, but try to maintain breath awareness.

Then you must merge and synchronize the mantra *soham* with the up and down movement of breath. Be simultaneously aware of both the rising and descending breath and the sound of *soham* made at the throat.

Mantra and breath must be synchronized so that:
So sounds with the upward moving inhalation.
Ham sounds with the downward moving exhalation.
There should be unceasing awareness of *soham* as you breathe in and out from the navel to the throat.

If your mind wanders, let it, but know that it is wandering. Maintain mantra and breath awareness.

Continue in this manner to the end of the time that you have assigned for practice.

Stage 2: Exactly the same practice as in stage 1 but with an emphasis on *hamso*.
Start with exhalation – *ham*
Finish with inhalation – *so*.

There should be no pauses between *ham* and *so*, but a slight pause after one round of *hamso*. That is, there should be no pause between exhalation and inhalation but a slight pause at the end of inhalation before exhaling.

Stage 3: Now the mantra *soham* is split so that you hear *so* with inhalation and *ham* with exhalation. That is, there is no continuity between *so* and *ham*. They are regarded as separate mantras without merging with each other. There should be a continuous cycle of *so* and *ham* with inhalation and exhalation respectively.

182

Stage 4: Same as stage 3, but now there should be continuous merging of *so* with *ham*. That is, on inhalation and exhalation, *so* and *ham* will repeat with continuous and endless cycle: *so-ham-so-ham-so-ham*. Another variation is: on the upward movement of breath (inhalation), *so* moves from the navel to the heart. The inhalation continues from the heart to the throat, but with the *ham*, exhalation begins from the throat with the breath moving downwards and the mantra *ham* continues. From the heart, the exhalation continues downward to the navel but with the mantra *so*. This is a continuous cycle with no beginning and no end. *Soham* merges with *hamso*.

Kundalini kriyas

These techniques are part of the practices of kriya yoga and have a powerful effect on the pranic body as well as the physical and mental bodies. They generate prana and bring about a realignment of the pranic and physical bodies. They act in the same way as a chiropractic manipulation but on the psychic and pranic levels of the human organism. For further details of these practices refer to *Meditations from the Tantras* by Swami Satyananda Saraswati, published by the Bihar School of Yoga.

Nada Sanchalana (conducting the sound consciousness)

Sit or lie in a comfortable position.
Close your eyes and become aware of breathing.
Do ujjayi pranayama, continuing breath awareness.
After a few minutes imagine that as you breathe in, your breath moves upwards in the spine passage from mooladhara chakra (at the perineum) to sahasrara chakra (crown of the head). As you breathe out, chant *om* loudly and feel the breath and *om* moving downwards in the spine from sahasrara to mooladhara.
This is one round. Complete thirteen rounds.
Practice note: the 'a' sound begins in sahasrara and the 'm' sound ends in mooladhara.

Pawan Sanchalana (conducting the breath consciousness)

This practice is very similar to nada sanchalana.

Sit or lie in a comfortable position.

Close your eyes.

As you breathe in, feel the breath moving upwards in the spine from mooladhara to sahasrara.

As you breathe out, feel the breath moving down the spine from sahasrara to mooladhara.

Do ujjayi pranayama throughout.

Complete 49 rounds.

Shabda Sanchalana (conducting the word consciousness)

This is the same as pawan sanchalana, but you must mentally feel the mantra *so* in conjunction with the breath rising up the spine as you breathe in, and the mantra *ham* descending in the spine as you exhale.

Ujjayi pranayama should be done throughout.

Complete 59 rounds.

Yoga Nidra

Yoga nidra is a systematic method of inducing complete mental, physical and emotional relaxation. It is a state of relaxed awareness on the border between sleep and wakefulness, allowing contact with the subconscious and unconscious minds.

Yoga nidra is the yogic tranquilizer, the natural means to establish harmony and wellbeing throughout the entire system. It is a superbly effective system of meditation and, for people who are sick or weak, it rejuvenates the nervous system, awakening prana and great healing power. Yoga nidra is especially useful in overcoming psychosomatic diseases, and similar techniques are used in clinics and hospitals throughout the world.

This technique can be practised anywhere, at any time. However, the best place is a well-ventilated room with soft lighting and a comfortable temperature. Clothing should be minimal and very loose, and a light sheet might be necessary to protect the practitioner from the cold or insects. Privacy is essential and interruptions should be avoided.

The best time to do yoga nidra is in the early morning, between four and six, or just before you go to sleep. Once you have chosen a time, try to stick to it. Do not practise immediately after eating; allow at least two hours for digestion of a heavy meal and an hour for the settling of light refreshments.

185

Yoga nidra is practised in the pose called *shavasana*, with the head, trunk and limbs in one straight line. However, some people will prefer to use a thin pillow under the head or under the small of the back.

You should aim during the practice to gain a grasp of the technique so that you can recall all the instructions without conscious effort. We recommend that you learn this technique from a yoga teacher, but if this is not possible, you could put the instructions on tape or have someone read them to you.

Resolve

The resolve is a short, positive phrase which is repeated at the beginning and end of the practice of yoga nidra. It is a seed that is planted deep in the subconscious mind and can bring astounding results if used with sincerity and feeling. The resolve has great healing potential, planting a positive suggestion at a time when the subconscious mind is in the state of greatest receptivity. It should be short, pointed and deeply felt. The following resolves are very useful:

- I will attain perfect health.
- I will become whole.
- I am unchanging consciousness, beyond disease.

You should continue to repeat your resolve, in exactly the same words, with a fervent and determined attitude, until it is a reality in your life.

Visualization

One of the most active areas of the brain is the visual cortex, indicating that the brain is very receptive to visual imagery. This means that inner or mental visualization has very powerful effects on the brain and thus the whole organism. In the following practice of yoga nidra we exploit this fact for self-healing by giving specific visualizations for hypertension.

At first these visualizations will require a lot of imagination, but with practise they will gain clarity and substance.

186

As your awareness expands you will not only move towards health but will also start to take off into the realms of higher consciousness.

Preparation: Get ready for yoga nidra. Lie in shavasana and make yourself as comfortable as possible. Keep your feet apart and let them flop a little sideways, arms close to the body with the palms upwards. *pause* Adjust your blanket, clothes and position so that you can practise yoga nidra without moving and without any physical discomfort. Please close your eyes and keep them closed. *long pause* The practice of yoga nidra is the act of hearing and the act of feeling, these are the only important factors. *pause* In yoga nidra you function at the level of awareness plus the level of listening. In dreams you have no control, in yoga nidra you are the creator of the dream. *pause* Say to yourself mentally, 'I am not going to sleep'...say firmly, 'I will not sleep'. *pause* Give yourself some time to become calm and steady...take a deep breath and as you breathe in feel calmness diffusing throughout the body. *pause* As you breathe out say to yourself mentally: "Relax".

Become aware of sounds in the distance, become aware of the most distant sounds that you can hear. *pause* Let your sense of hearing operate just like a radar beam...searching out any distant sounds and following them for a few seconds. *pause* Move your attention quickly from sound to sound...without attempting to identify the source. *pause* Gradually bring your attention to closer sounds...to sounds outside this building...and then to sounds inside the building. *pause* Now develop your awareness of this room...without opening your eyes visualize the four walls, the ceiling, the floor, your body lying on the floor. *pause* Become aware of the existence of your physical body lying on the floor...total awareness of your body lying in perfect stillness. *pause* Your body lying on the floor...develop awareness of the

187

meeting points between your body and the floor.

Become aware of the natural breath...be very aware of the deep, natural, spontaneous breath. Do not concentrate for this will interfere with the natural process. *pause* Keep on listening and know that you are breathing. *pause* The practice of yoga nidra begins now...say mentally to yourself: 'I am going to practise yoga nidra. I will not sleep. I will not sleep. I am going to practise yoga nidra'.

Resolve: This is the time to make your resolve. *pause* A simple resolve. Please state your resolve with feeling and awareness three times. Nothing trivial, but a positive goal for whole being. *pause*.

Rotation of consciousness: Rotation of consciousness through the different centres of the body. As quickly as possible your awareness is to jump from point to point. Repeat mentally the name of each part and simultaneously become aware of that part. The practice always begins with the right hand...

Right side: Right hand thumb, second finger, third finger, fourth finger, fifth finger, palm, wrist, elbow, shoulder, armpit, waist, hip, right thigh, knee, calf muscle, ankle, heel, sole, right big toe, second toe, third toe, fourth toe, fifth toe...

Left side: Left hand thumb, second finger, third finger, fourth finger, fifth finger, palm, wrist, elbow, shoulder, armpit, waist, hip, left thigh, knee, calf muscle, ankle, heel, sole, left big toe, second toe, third toe, fourth toe, fifth toe...

Back: Right shoulder, left shoulder, right shoulder blade, left shoulder blade...right buttock, left buttock, the spine...the whole of the back together...

Front: Top of the head, forehead, right eyebrow, left eyebrow, the space between the eyebrows, right eye, left eye, right ear, left ear, right cheek, left cheek, nose, tip of the nose, upper lip, lower lip, chin, throat, right collarbone, left collarbone, right chest, left chest, middle of the chest, navel, abdomen, lower abdomen...

Major parts: Whole of the right leg, whole of the left leg, both legs together...Whole of the right arm, whole of the left arm, both arms together...Whole of the back, whole of the front, whole of the head...together...whole body...whole body...whole body. *long pause*

Breathing: Draw your attention to the natural ingoing and outgoing breath. *pause* Feel the breath move along the passage between the navel and the throat...on inhalation it rises from the navel to the throat, on exhalation it descends from the throat to the navel. *pause* Be completely aware of the respiration, navel to throat, throat to navel...do not try to force the breath...just awareness. *pause* Now, as you breathe in, feel the body expand, and as you breathe out, feel the body relax...inhale and relax the body with healing energy...exhale and expand, feeling the impurities flow out of your system on the breath. *pause* Inhale and expand as the prana flows to every cell and every fibre of the body...exhale and relax, washing away negativity and impurities. *pause* Do not sleep but continue the practice. *long pause*

Visualization: Are you awake or are you sleeping? Check yourself and say mentally 'I am awake'... Become aware of manipura chakra, the psychic centre in the solar plexus region. Manipura chakra, in the spinal cord behind the navel...As you exhale, feel the vital energy in your body gathering in manipura chakra. *pause* Exhale and withdraw all your prana, all your healing life-force, into manipura chakra. *pause* Then as you inhale, feel this healing energy streaming to all parts of your body. *pause* See the prana as streaks of light converging on manipura as you exhale...then as you inhale, visualize this healing prana flaring out from manipura to all parts of your body, like golden, healing sunrays. *pause* See a brilliant sun, a gold fiery sun at your navel, pulsing with health-giving energy. *pause* Just as from a charcoal fire you see sparks shooting out with a hissing noise, so you see the healing energies moving in your body...clearly

189

see luminous shafts of energy...like the iridescent light streaks streaming forth from fireworks. *pause* Imagine manipura to be a storehouse of infinite light streaks...it is like a volcano erupting light particles that move with white-lightning speed...they permeate the whole body. *pause* Then the eruption stops and the lightning withdraws to the source, to reappear at the next explosion...volcano of bright healing prana. *long pause*

Healing symbols: Now take your awareness to chidakasha, concentrate on the space you see in front of your closed eyes. *pause* In this space you see a blue sky...a giant golden sun...the warmth and the golden energy of this sun...an explosion of light...a blue sky...a cross...a six pointed star...a garden with a circular pool at the centre...in the pool a fountain...from the fountain a fine spray of golden, life-giving liquid...blue lotus...white lotus...red lotus...shiva lingam...a candle flame...a golden egg...stars at night...golden harvest moon...a golden river...a sea of golden liquid...an endless golden ocean...see your self at the edge of this ocean...you dive into the sea...feel it surround every part of your body...refreshing, tingling...soaking to the very depths of your being...recharging your whole body with vitality...smooth feeling...see yourself diving to the depths of the ocean...deep...towards a shining, green jewel...hold this sea emerald...gaze into the green jewel...it explodes in a blaze of light and you find yourself on the shore. *long pause*

Inner space: Bring your awareness back to chidakasha, bring your awareness back to the dark space you see before your closed eyes. *pause* Watch the darkness that you see very carefully, with detachment, do not become involved. *pause* Rest your mind in this warm and friendly darkness...if any subtle phenomena manifest, for example, colours or patterns, simply take note of these and continue with your awareness. *pause* If thoughts occur let them come and go, do not interfere or become involved in the mental disturbances which may occur but continue to watch the dark space, with complete awareness. *long pause*

Resolve: Your resolve, remember your resolve. Repeat the same resolve you made at the beginning of the practice in the same words and with the same attitude. Repeat your resolve with feeling and emphasis three times. *pause*

Finish: Become aware of your breathing, become aware of your natural breath. *pause* Awareness of breathing... and awareness of relaxation. *pause* Develop awareness of relaxation and awareness of your physical existence. *pause* Become aware of your arms and legs and your body lying stretched out on the floor. *pause*
Develop awareness of the room, walls ceiling...noises in the room and noises outside...bring your mind out... become completely external. *pause* Lie quietly for a few moments keeping your eyes closed. Start moving your body, stretch yourself slowly...do not hurry. *pause* When you are sure that you are wide awake, sit up slowly and open your eyes. The practice of yoga nidra is now complete.

Om Tat Sat

Alternative visualization

This visualization may be inserted in the above practice to replace the section 'healing symbols'. It is specifically directed at channelling the healing energies of the body to correct the deficiency in the blood vessels.

Now send the golden light from manipura to the heart...you can feel the energy travel from your navel to your heart...and feel the warmth. *pause* The heart starts to glow with golden light...with each throb of the heart the light grows more intense...with each beat the energy gathers into a sphere of light...inside the heart...you can see this energy becoming more intense, golden, and you

191

can feel the warmth...from the centre of your body where your heart is. *pause* You can feel the energy travel from the heart like a comet trailing a tail of golden kite. *pause* First into the head...every blood vessel is now suffused with warm, golden light...which has changed the very nature of the blood and made it look golden. *pause* This golden energy pervades the length of the blood vessels...into the muscles surrounding the vessels...into the cells of the body which are glowing with this golden energy. *pause* Now see every blood vessel of the head slowly melting and dissolving because of the heat of this golden light...dissolving into a cast made by the light...the form of the vessels is there, but the tissue has dissolved...the blood is still flowing through this channel. *pause* As each vessel dissolves into the golden form, all the impurities and tensions have been dissolved and purged from the system...the prana has dissolved away the impurities and left only pure, warm, tingling energy. *pause* Now see the golden light fading and the vessels reforming...the same place, but new vessels carry the blood. *pause* Follow the prana back to the heart...it moves from the heart into both arms and the same process of melting takes place...watch this process. *pause* The light moves into the blood vessels, charging the blood, purifying, and then moves into the tissues melting...golden form is all that remains. *pause* Now watch as the blood carries prana through the trunk, into the legs...throughout the whole body. *pause* The whole body is purified and glows with golden light...the whole body...whole body...whole body...whole body glowing with golden, healing light. *long pause*.

For full details of these practices consult the publications: *Asana Pranayama Mudra Bandha* published by Bihar Yoga Bharati; *Meditations from the Tantras* and *Yoga Nidra* published by Bihar School of Yoga.

Appendices

Low Blood Pressure

This chapter on low blood pressure, or hypotension, has been added to complete the spectrum of problems that can occur with disturbance of the blood pressure regulating mechanisms. Many people are confused as to what constitutes low blood pressure, especially when it comes to contemplating treatment.

What is low blood pressure?

The term low blood pressure is used to describe the situation where blood pressure falls below that which is normal for a certain age. Once again, as for high blood pressure, it is difficult to give an exact definition of what constitutes low blood pressure because every individual is different and will react differently in various situations. There are two main situations in which low blood pressure comes to light.

1. *The first* occurs when a routine physical examination reveals, in an otherwise healthy adult, a blood pressure of say 100/60 or less. In this situation the doctor will usually measure and compare the blood pressure while the patient is standing and lying. Any difference between the two will highlight instability of the autonomic nervous system and its inability to adequately adjust the body to the normal or stressful demands placed on it. People whose standing and lying blood pressures are equal, are usually those whose pressures lie within the lower range of normal

195

and who will go through life without trouble. In one sense, they are lucky because a lower blood pressure places less stress and strain on their internal organs.

2. *The second group* are those who suffer from the symptoms of low blood pressure, which usually occur on suddenly standing up from a lying or seated position. These symptoms can range from weakness, light headedness, nausea and a sinking feeling in the upper abdomen, to fainting and loss of consciousness, usually for a few seconds or minutes, but occasionally longer. Fainting is also called syncope.

What is the cause of those symptoms?

From the yogic point of view, the symptoms of low blood pressure occur because of imbalance in an autonomic nervous system weakened by mental tension and improper lifestyle. This lowers the prana shakti, adversely affecting the functioning of our physical body.

From the physiological point of view there are two main causes of syncope or fainting, both of which are due to reflex peripheral vasodilation of blood vessels in the abdomen and skin which in turn leads to pooling of blood in the extremities and a consequent reduction in the amount of blood reaching the brain:

1. *Vasovagal attacks* which are usually caused by an emotional disturbance, such as fear, disgust or surprise, for example, at the sight of blood or an accident. Pain, lack of food, hot atmospheres and prolonged standing commonly pre-dispose to it. The subject of the attack becomes pale and clammy; the blood pressure and heart rate are low. The individual in this situation should be left in a comfortable lying position so that blood can flow into the brain and the attack should then quickly subside by itself.

2. *Postural hypotension* occurs commonly in elderly patients suffering or recovering from an illness. Certain drugs can also cause this as an unwanted side effect. It usually occurs on standing up suddenly, or while standing too

long, especially in a hot atmosphere. Soldiers standing on parade often faint because of this.

The symptoms of low blood pressure can also occur in patients suffering from high blood pressure. They may take too much hypertensive medication or they may be weak after an acute illness or be in a hot stuffy atmosphere. Patients with a normally raised blood pressure of 220/110 or even 160/110 may experience symptoms of low blood pressure with a so-called normal blood pressure of 120/80. This means that 120/80 is low for them. Their bodies have acclimatized to a higher than normal blood pressure and, especially if they are suffering from hardening of the arteries (arteriosclerosis), they require this high blood pressure to push nutrients and oxygen into their tissues. A lowering of blood pressure can be catastrophic, causing a mild or even severe stroke. Therefore, when we talk about low blood pressure, we have to relate it to a person's age, individual and physical condition.

There are other more serious causes of hypotension, such as in certain heart conditions and anaemia, and all people suffering from any unusual, undiagnosed symptoms are well advised to have a proper physical examination by a qualified physician.

How should we treat hypotension?

As for hypertension, there are is no reliable medical way of treating hypotension. Of course, any underlying disease or weakness should be medically treated and the body strengthened by adequate diet and rest. However, often symptoms persist and these are best handled by a few simple yogic practices which revolve around surya namaskara, nadi shodhana and bhastrika pranayama. Asana and pranayama should be performed twice a day for the best effect: asana and pranayama in the morning, a few simple asana before dinner and nadi shodhana and yoga nidra before sleep. A typical yogic regime for hypotension would start off with pawanmuktasana part 1, nadi shodhana and bhastrika pranayama and yoga nidra. This would help to gradually strengthen the body, remove underlying imbalance in the autonomic nervous system (especially by nadi shodhana) and also aid in convalescence.

After a few weeks of the above regime or in otherwise healthy people, asanas such as pawanmuktasana part 2, shakti bandha series, surya namaskara and dynamically performed major asana, such as paschimottanasana, dhanurasana and ardha matsyendrasana can be added. After some time more vigorous asana such as mayurasana, yoga mudra and chakrasana can be included as the individual becomes more adept.

Bhastrika pranayama powerfully strengthens and balances a weakened autonomic nervous system. Surya bheda pranayama can occasionally be used under expert guidance. Kunjal and neti are also often used to cleanse the body and strengthen the nervous system.

Inverted asana and the overuse of static postures should be avoided. All practices, of course, should be learned under expert guidance so that the nervous system can be initially relaxed, then balanced and strengthened in a progressive, systematic manner. In this way, people suffering from symptoms of low blood pressure, or any disease for that matter, can slowly but surely regain their birthright of good health and an active, happy life.

Suggestions for Diet

Diet plays a major role in the alleviation of hypertension. Medical and yogic treatment will help bring down your blood pressure, but in order to maintain this you must revise your diet. The following suggestions are provided to give the basic outline your should follow in order to bring your blood pressure down to the desired level.

The basis of this regime is a low salt, vegetarian diet with a moderate number of calories. This has the threefold effect of lowering blood pressure, reducing weight and increasing overall health. Please remember that we are only making suggestions for your better health, but you must apply them to your individual situation with a certain degree of common sense. Do not become fanatical about what you eat, because this will only create more tension. Slowly begin to incorporate the yogic pattern of eating into your lifestyle, step by step, in an aware and relaxed way. You will not be blindly accepting a doctrine, but will be gaining knowledge that will increase your body awareness and your health.

We have found through our experience that a vegetarian diet is the most conducive to good health and yogic living. Research is implicating meat in such diseases as hypertension, colonic cancer, heart attack and certain joint diseases, to name but a few. Meat is also the main source of saturated fatty acids and cholesterol, thought to play a role in hardening of the arteries and subsequent increase in blood pressure.

199

There are many arguments in favour of a vegetarian diet but not everyone wants to stop eating meat. Certain types of meat have been found to be better for you than others. These are the 'white' meats, so called because of their absence of blood, including breast of chicken, non-fatty fish, and veal. If you find a vegetarian diet too demanding then at least try to eat these meats.

There are times when we may have to break a vegetarian diet, even if we have adopted this for ourselves. Certain social occasions may demand that we eat something we do not like so as not to offend our host. However, we should keep in mind that if we have healthy habits as the basis of our lifestyle, the occasional indiscretion will do no harm. It is what we eat every day that decides whether we become sick or remain healthy.

Diet for hypertension

Probably the most important aspect of diet for the hypertensive person is a low salt, low fat content. Less salt on its own is the more important of the two and will in itself help to reduce your blood pressure. This means that no salt should be added to cooking and none at the table.

Instead of adding salt to your cooking, add spices or herbs. They do wonders for increasing flavour and taste. To enhance flavour do what we do here at Bihar School of Yoga, Munger, India. Food is first lightly fried in a little vegetable oil and then water is added to complete the cooking. In this way you get a good balance of unsaturated fatty acids, essential for good health, and cholesterol in the correct quantity. The food is neither greasy nor tasteless, especially if herbs are added. Taste is enhanced and health maintained.

Other methods of preparation, except deep frying, should offer a wide enough range of alternatives so that you can cut down on salts and fats. All food should be raw, grilled, baked or steamed, but not fried. You may be able to go without breakfast and this should help. Eat at regular times and in small quantities, rather than overeating. An ashram diet tends to rebalance one's weight and keeps fat and salt to a minimum. It mainly consists of:

- vegetables (sauteed first then boiled)
- split peas, lentils, chickpeas (dahl)
- chapatis (unleavened wholewheat bread)
- rice
- fruit and raw vegetables

This diet balances the complete requirement of vitamins, minerals, protein, carbohydrates and fat in order to maintain health at the optimum level. Neither does it demand extra energy to digest nor does it add toxins. In fact, it is a cleansing diet that leaves us feeling satisfied and well-nourished. On this basis you can add the occasional indulgence, such as sweets and so on, but do not make these a regular habit.

Avoid all foods which contain:

1. *Salt*, such as tinned, cured and bottled meats, foods with preservatives added, sauces, and so on.
2. *Bicarbonate of soda*, such as in biscuits and cakes.
3. *Excess fats*, such as fried foods, butter, margarine, dripping, cooking fat, lard, fatty meats and fish (goose, duck, pork, bacon, herring, kippers, sardines and salmon), egg yolk, cream, ice cream, pastries, cakes, chocolate, and so on.

Reducing fat and obesity

It is a fact that some people, who have a slower metabolism, can put on weight more easily than most others. However, we only get fat if we overeat. By following the suggestions in the preceding sections it is possible to reduce both excess fat and cholesterol and to reduce body weight. This happens quite naturally when we undertake yogic discipline.

To aid the process of weight reduction eat mainly raw fruits, vegetables and split peas. Avoid excessive carbohydrates, sugar (in any form) and fats, for example, white bread, cakes, milk, cream, cheese, (except low fat cottage cheese), jam, dried fruit, alcoholic beverages, and so on.

Balancing the diet

When you have finally sorted out your own individual 'should' and 'should nots', then you can begin to adapt yourself to your new regime. When you cook, prepare your food with care and awareness and you will feel the difference in taste. If you then eat in a relaxed and comfortable atmosphere, with good companions, the flavour and pranic content is increased even more. Rushing an inadequate meal only serves to increase sympathetic stimulation further. By relaxing, however, we turn on the parasympathetic component, the digestive juices are balanced, and awareness is heightened. This will automatically turn down the sympathetic overstimulation and lower the blood pressure.

The Pillars of Life

Clairvoyants see the pranic body as a coloured, luminous cloud or aura around the physical body, like the sun flaring from behind the eclipsing moon. Kirlian photography may have captured this effect and made a normally invisible aspect of our being visible to us all. The pranic body is made up of nadis carrying energy, organized around the three most important and central nadis: ida, pingala and sushumna. The physical body corresponds to this layout as it is vitally interconnected with the pranic body which supplies the current and power to make this body-machine work. It is prana which energizes and pervades every aspect of mind, metabolism, and sensory functioning.

When you open up the abdomen of a person while he is on the operating table it is possible to see the blood vessels pulsating. The arteries and veins stand out clearly from each other even though they lie side by side. Alongside the spinal cord the main vessels are seen carrying blood to and from the heart. On the left side the aorta carries blood downward from the heart, while on the right of the spinal cord the inferior vena cava is carrying the blood up to the heart. Just so, the ida nadi flows on the left side of the pranic body and the pingala nadi flows on the right. In between flows sushumna nadi, the spiritual channel, the middle path. Ida and pingala represent the dual aspects of nature. Ida represents female, yin, cold, passive, matter, moon, imagination, negativity, and the metal silver. Pingala represents male, yang, hot, active, energy, sun, dynamism, positivity and the metal gold. Sushumna is the ideal state of balance and synthesis of both and is known as the middle way or 'royal road'

With insight gained through yoga, the circulatory system is perceived as being a reflection of the pranic body's network of nadis. The arteries correspond to pingala nadi in that they are outgoing from the heart, red, dynamic, feed the body and regulate body warmth. The veins correspond to ida nadi in that they travel to the heart, are blue, passive, take away wastes from the cells of the body, and are not concerned with body heat regulation. As the connecting link between the polarity of arteries and veins, the heart and capillaries represent sushumna, the middle way.

On the physical level the active, dynamic component of the circulatory system (the arteries) are on the left of the central spinal cord, while the veins (the passive and receptive component) lie on the right. The sushumna nadi lies within the spinal cord between the arterial and venous network.

To grasp the concept of the interdependence of ida, pingala and sushumna we must imagine a point. This is the point before creation. Imagine that you have split this point in two and drawn the poles apart. There are now three components: at one extreme is ida, at the other pingala, and in between is sushumna. Yet they are all one continuum. This symbolic representation works both at the macrocosmic level of the universe and at the microcosmic level of our body. Within the twenty-four hour daily revolution of the earth lies the dark-light cycle. Within the twelve month revolution of the sun lie the hot and cold seasons. Within the physical body lie the arteries and veins that comprise the circulatory system. This dual system is to be seen in all things merely as opposite poles of the one whole.

In yogic philosophy it is stated that to open the sushumna and thereby reach higher consciousness we must balance ida and pingala. That is, we must balance mind and body, work and rest, inner awareness with outer awareness, and all aspects of our lives. There we harmonize and balance our microcosm with the macrocosm, and we tune in to the deeper spheres of true understanding.

Understanding is achieved in meditation, and the process of evolution of the microcosm within the macrocosm proceeds. This evolution of man is represented also in the inner body processes. The movement of blood from and to the heart has its reflection in the spiritual journey. In the macrocosm, man is moving from his original state of oneness with the universe, through the process of differentiation into myriads of individual and ego-conscious minds, and then back towards his original unitive state. The microcosm in each individual artery starts from the one, the heart. It branches, multiplies and divides endlessly, becoming smaller and more separate from its original union. We are all capillaries of the divine energy if we desire and turn our attention to the source of our creation.

When we expand our consciousness to the level of sushumna we become aware of unity, that the duality is one. This is attained by balancing ida and pingala. This balances our autonomic nervous system and cures hypertension.

Internal Organs

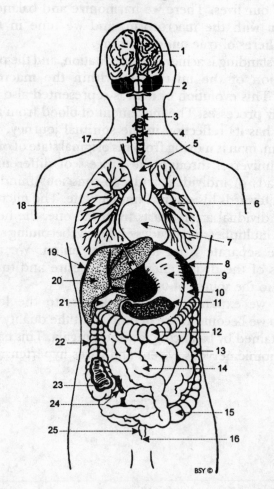

BSY ©

1. Brain	10. Spleen	18. Right Lung
2. Spinal cord	11. Pancreas	19. Diaphragm
3. Vertebral column	12. Transverse colon	20. Liver
4. Trachea	(large intestine)	21. Gall Bladder
5. Aorta	13. Descending colon	22. Ascending colon
6. Left Lung	14. Small intestine	23. Cecum
7. Heart	15. Sigmoid colon	24. Appendix
8. Diaphragm	16. Anus	25. Rectum
9. Stomach	17. Oesophagus	

Glossary

Acute – when referring to disease it means having a short and relatively severe course.

Adrenal gland – two endocrine glands situated on top of the outer cortex and inner medulla. The former secretes cortisone, the latter, adrenaline.

Adrenaline – a hormone secreted by the adrenal medulla in response to nervous stimulation or lowered blood sugar. It contracts the blood vessels, raises blood pressure, stimulates the heart and prepares the body for intense muscular activity and stress.

Adrenocorticotrophic hormone (ACTH) – a pituitary hormone that stimulates the adrenal glands to release cortisone.

Allopathy – the popular modern medical system which cures by using substances incompatible with or antagonistic to the condition which is to be cured or alleviated.

Alpha rhythm – brain waves which beat at a rate of 8-13 cycles per second and which indicate relaxation, preliminary states of meditation, receptivity to ESP, and spontaneous, creative states of mind.

Amphetamines – central nervous system stimulants that increase blood pressure.

Anahata chakra – the psychic centre at the heart associated with the element air, the lungs, the heart and compassion. It has twelve petals and its beeja mantra is *yam*.

207

Angina pectoris – cramping pains in the centre of the chest caused by hardening of the arteries of the heart.

Aorta – main artery arising directly from the heart.

Apana – one of the five manifestations of prana in the human body. It is associated with outgoing breath; it is situated below the navel and controls excretion of urine and faeces, and the expulsion of the foetus at birth.

Archetype – original model, prototype.

Arterioles – small arteries which control the direction of blood flow and its distribution to internal organs.

Artery – blood vessel carrying blood from the heart.

Arteriosclerosis – hardening of the arteries due to the deposition of fat and protein, which eventually leads to blockage of the vessel and death of the tissues.

Asana – a steady or comfortable posture.

Atrium – upper chamber of the heart. There are two, left and right.

Aura – subtle emanation; the atmosphere attending a person.

Autonomic nervous system – part of the nervous system which controls the body's internal environment automatically, though it can be regulated by willpower.

Barbiturates – drugs used for their tranquilizing effects, especially in psychosis, (today no longer believed to be safe because of their addictive properties).

Bhagavad Gita – the great Indian text taken from the epic 'The Mahabharata', in which Lord Krishna gives Arjuna instructions in yoga.

Biofeedback – a scientific technique utilizing machines to detect when the body is relaxed or performing a predetermined task, and then to relay the information back to the conscious awareness of the subject.

Biorhythms – the cyclical rhythms of the body which harmonize with the natural environment in terms of light-dark cycles, moon phases, etc.

Blood – the fluid that circulates through the heart, arteries, capillaries and veins, carrying nutrients and oxygen to the cells, and taking away waste products.

Blood/brain barrier – the membrane barrier protecting the brain and selectively absorbing oxygen and sugar.

Brahmamuhurta – the time between four and six a.m. This is the sattwic time of day, best suited to yogic sadhana.

Brain waves – electrical emanations from the brain; detected on an electroencephalogram (EEG), which is a very sensitive voltmeter.

Capillary – a minute blood vessel, the thickness of a hair, which connects arterioles to venules.

Carbon dioxide – an odourless, colourless gas, formed in the body tissues and eliminated mainly via the lungs.

Cardiac muscle – heart muscle.

Cardiac output – the amount of blood pumped by the heart over a given length of time.

Cardiovascular system – the heart and blood vessels.

Carotid sinus – the dilated portion of the carotid artery which is stimulated by pressure changes in the blood system and reports to the brain.

Cells – the living, active basis of plant and animal tissue: composed of protoplasm and mucus within a membrane.

Cervical – pertaining to the neck.

Chakras – psychic energy centres.

Chronic – persisting over a long period of time.

Cortex (cortical) – the external layer.

Diastole – the period of dilation of the heart.

Electrocardiogram – a voltmeter which is arranged so as to allow one to picture the action of the heart.

Endocrine glands – a group of organs which secrete hormones directly into the blood. This system controls metabolism and the internal environment, as well as affecting mind, personality and emotions.

Feedback – the return of information to its source.

Galvanic skin resistance (GSR) – a measurement of the electrical conductance of the skin which varies with sweat production. The greater the GSR the greater the relaxation.

Gastric – pertaining to the stomach.

Gene – the biological unit of heredity, self-reproducing and located on a definite part of a chromosome.

Heart – chest muscle which maintains the blood circulation.

Heredity – the genetic transmission of a particular quality or trait from parent to offspring.

Hormone – a chemical substance, usually secreted by endocrine glands, to regulate the activity of various organs.

Hypertension – hyper-tenseness; persistently high arterial blood pressure, categorized as follows:

• *essential*: hypertension with no known cause.

• *labile*: not persistent; blood pressure rises with increased tension and stress.

• *malignant*: an accelerated, severe hypertensive condition with poor prognosis.

Hypertrophy – overgrowth.

Hypo – beneath, under, deficient.

Hypometabolic – a state of body function where cell activity is lessened, thus requiring less food, oxygen, etc. Less energy is consumed in the body, leaving more for the mind.

Hypothalamus – an important section of the midbrain which exercises control over the major organs of the body.

Ida – one of the three main nadis in the human body.

Idiopathic – unknown cause, self-originated.

Immune system – renders us resistant to disease.

Inferior vena cava (IVC) – the major vein that brings blood back to the heart from the legs and trunk.

Jivatma – individual embodied spirit.

Kirlian photography – system of high voltage electrical photography that has revealed hitherto unseen energies in the body.

Kundalini – the coiled power at the base of the spine; shakti; cosmic energy.

Lactate – the substance produced by the muscles from oxidation of glycogen.

Manipura – the navel chakra associated with fire, the digestive system and strength.

210

Meditation – dhyana, inner consciousness, one-pointed awareness.

Medulla – the central part of an organ, e.g. the adrenal medulla.

Medulla oblongata – the lowest part of the brain that is attached to the spinal cord. It governs breathing, the circulation and special senses.

Melatonin – hormone secreted by the pineal gland which enhances immune activity and slows the ageing process.

Metabolism – the combined processes of building up and breaking down of substances in the body.

Nadi – flow of prana and chitta.

Neural – pertaining to the nervous system.

Neuro-endocrinal axis – the coordination between the nervous and endocrine systems.

Neurone – a conducting nerve cell; the basic unit of the nervous system.

Neurosis – conflict of energies within the mind; creates short circuits and chaos in brain action and structure; reduces flexibility of personality and activity.

Noradrenaline – a hormone secreted by the medulla of the adrenal glands.

Obesity – excess fat in the body.

Ojas – spiritual energy, generated by control over the pranic systems of the body, especially sexual energy.

Oxygen – a gaseous element essential to metabolism.

Palpitations – unduly rapid action of the heart which is noted by the patient to be regular or irregular.

Parapsychology – a new science to investigate psychic and related phenomena not accepted or studied by modern psychology, such as ESP, pranic healing and acupuncture.

Parasympathetic – the part of the autonomic nervous system concerned with relaxation, rest and play activity.

Peripheral resistance – the amount of resistance met by the blood as it flows into the peripheral arterioles. In part, it is dependent on the degree of constriction of the blood vessels.

Pingala – one of the three main nadis in the human body.

Plasma – fluid portion of the blood in which the cells are suspended.

Prana – the universal, cosmic energy or force that gives life to all things; the manifestation of this force in the human vehicle. Also, prana is one of the five subdivisions of cosmic prana, extending in the body from the diaphragm to the throat.

Pranamaya kosha – the vital body of prana, one of the five sheaths of the human vehicle.

Pranayama – control of prana; as well as of breath; breathing exercises.

Premature ventricular contraction (PVC) – a cardiac arrhythmic or uneven beating of the heart.

Psychic healing – healing through the direction of prana to the site of disease.

Psychosomatic disease – disease caused by psychological stress.

Pulmonary circulation – blood travelling from the heart to the lungs and back.

Raja yoga – Patanjali's system of yoga, the eight aspects of which are yama; niyama; asana; pranayama; pratyahara; dharana; dhyana; samadhi.

Relaxation – the opposite of contraction, tension; a state of restful awareness and alertness.

Respiratory system – mainly the lungs, trachea and nose; the system concerned with gases - the intake of oxygen and exhalation of carbon dioxide and wastes.

Reticular activating system (RAS) – an important nervous junction mainly in the brain stem, concerned with arousal, alertness, sleep, emotional expression, regulation of posture, muscle tone and visceral reactions.

Sadhana – spiritual practice.

Samana – one of the five manifestations of prana in the body, extending from the navel to the heart.

Samskaras – accumulated mental impressions and tendencies that are a residue of past experience.

Sankalpa – a resolve or promise to oneself, embedded in the subconscious mind and repeated continuously so that it becomes a reality.

Serotonin – a neuro-transmitter linked with circuits of the brain which utilize emotional responses.

Shakti – a name for prana, cosmic energy.

Sushumna – the most important nadi in the body, running down the centre of the spinal chord.

Sinus node – a collection of atypical heart muscle fibres at the junction of the superior vena cava and the right atrium; the seat of the soul at a higher level.

Skeletal muscle – muscles used to move the bones; striped muscle, under conscious control.

Smooth muscle – muscle controlled by the autonomic nervous system, not readily accessible to conscious control.

Sphygmomanometer – an instrument to measure blood pressure.

Stress – the pull between opposites; constraining or compelling force; effort; demand on energy.

Superior vena cava (SVC) – the major vein draining blood from the head, arms and upper chest into the right atrium.

Sympathetic nervous system – that part of the autonomic nervous system used to prepare the body to handle stress and the 'fight or flight' reaction.

Symptoms – those subjective sensations or physical ailments that cause a patient to seek a doctor.

Systemic circulation – the blood travelling from the heart to the body cells; carrying oxygen away from the heart, and carbon dioxide and wastes back to the heart.

Systole – the time of active contraction of heart muscle.

Tension – stretching, being stretched, mental strain or excitement; a neurotic or abnormal response by the body to a stressful situation.

Thoracic – pertaining to the chest.

Tranquilizer – a drug which calms or quietens the nervous system without affecting clarity of consciousness.

Udana – one of the five manifestations of prana, extending from the throat to the crown of the head.

Vasoconstrictors – nerves which, if stimulated, constrict the blood vessels.

Vasodilators – nerves which, if stimulated, dilate the blood vessels.

Vasomotor system – the nervous subsystem which controls the dilation and constriction of blood vessels.

Vegetative system – those parts of the body controlled by the autonomic nervous system such as the lungs, blood vessels, intestines, and so on.

Vein – a blood vessel taking blood to the heart.

Ventricles – the lower chambers of the heart, of which there are two, right and left.

Vertebra – any one of the thirty-three bones of the spinal column.

Viscious circle – the sequence of events which leads up to progressively worse effects for the individual.

Virtuous circle – the sequence of events which leads up to better health and increased happiness.

Vyana – one of the five manifestations of prana, pervading the whole body.

References

Chapter 1

1 R.K. Wallace & H. Benson, 'Physiology of Meditation', *Scientific American*, vol. 226, no. 2, February 1972, pp.84–90.

R.K. Wallace, H. Benson, A.F. Wilson, M. Garret, 'Decreased Lactate During Transcendental Meditation', *Proceedings of the Federation of American Society for Experimental Biology*, vol. 30, no. 2, March–April 1971, p.376.

W.E. Huckabee, 'Relationships of Pyruvate and Lactate during Anaerobic Metabolism', *Journal of Clinical Investigation*, vol. 37, 1958, pp.224–254.

2 M. Friedman & R.H. Rosenman, *Type A Behaviour and Your Heart*, Knopf, New York, 1974.

3 *Ibid*

4 E. Gellhorn & W.F. Kiely, 'Autonomic Nervous System in Psychiatric Disorders', *Biological Psychiatry*, Joseph Mendels (ed), New York, John Wiley and Sons, 1973, ch. 11, pp.235–263.

5 D. Orme–Johnson, 'Autonomic Stability and Transcendental Meditation', *Psychosomatic Medicine*, vol. 35, no. 4, July–August 1973, pp.341–349.

6 D. Funkenstein, 'The Physiology of Fear and Anger', *Scientific American*, May 1955.

7 W. Tiller, 'Consciousness, Radiation and the Developing Sensory System', *The Dimensions of Healing, a Symposium*, (Transcript from the Academy of Parapsychology and Medicine), 1972, pp.61–85.

[8] E.E. Van Bount, et al., 'Penetration of Light into the Brains of Mammals', *Annals of New York Academy of Science*, 117, 1964, pp.217–224.

[9] K.S. Gopal, V. Anantharaman, S.D. Nishith, O.P. Bhatnagar, 'The Effects of Yogasanas on Muscular Tone and Cardiorespiratory Adjustments', *Yoga Life*, May 1975, pp.3–11.

Chapter 2

[10] Prof. L.K. White, 'International Comparison of Medical Care', *Scientific American*, vol. 233, no.2, August 1975.

[11] T. Pasek & W. Romanowski, 'Relaxation-Concentration Yoga Exercises in Current Physical Education', *FIEP Bulletin*, vol. 41, no. 3, July–September 1971, pp.90–92.

[12] Ibid, p.91.

[13] T. Pasek, W. Romanowski, et al. 'Studies on Physiological and Psychological Evaluation of the Yoga System of Exercises', *Wych. Fiz-Sport*, 1969, 3. pp.139–170.

[14] Vinekar Kuvalayananda, *Yogic Therapy – Its Basic Principles and Methods*, Ministry of Health, Govt. of India, New Delhi, 1963.

[15] K.S. Gopal, et al., op. cit., pp.3–11.

[16] R.K. Wallace & H. Benson, op. cit., p.81.

[17] K.S. Gopal, et al., op. cit., p.9.

[18] 'Electronic Evidence of auras, chakras in UCLA study', *Brain Mind Bulletin*, vol. 3, no. 9, March 20, 1978.

[19] 'Rumanians develop dynamic Kirlian-type process', *Brain Mind Bulletin*, vol. 3, no. 10, April 3, 1978.

[20] H. Motoyama, 'Hypnosis, Psychosis and Religious Experience', *IARP*, Research for Religion and Parapsychology, December 1976, vol. 2, no. 2, p.4.

[21] Patanjali Yoga Institute, Hyderabad, India, Quarterly Progress Report for the Quarter Ending September 30, 1972.

[22] K.K. Datey, S.N. Deshmukh, C.P. Dalvi, (late) S.L. Vinekar, 'Shavasana – A Yogic Exercise in the Management of Hypertension', *Angiology*, 20: pp.325–333, 1969.

[23] Ibid, p.333.

[24] Dr. D. David, *National Tatler*, June 24, 1973.

[25] Dr. D. Shapiro, et al., 'Effects of Feedback and Reinforcement on the Control of Human Systolic Blood Pressure', *Science*, 1969, 163, pp.588–590.

[26] J. Brener & R. Kleinman, 'Learned Control of Decrease in Systolic Blood Pressure', *Nature*, 1970, 226, p.1063.

[27] A. Christy & J. Vitale, 'Operant Conditioning of High Blood Pressure: A Pilot Study.(unpublished manuscript, San Francisco Veteran Admin. Hospital, 1971) from the book *Biofeedback: Turning on the Powers of Your Mind*, by M. Karlins & L.M. Andrews, Abacus, 1973, p.28.

[28] G. Luce & E. Peper, 'Biofeedback: Mind over Body, Mind over Mind', *New York Times Magazine*, 12/9/71. p.136.

[29] T. Weiss & B. Engel, 'Operant Conditioning of Heart Rate in Premature Ventricular Contractions', *Psychosomatic Medicine*, 1971, 33, p.391.

[30] G. Luce & E. Peper, op.cit, p.134.

[31] Dr. H.C. Patel, *The Lancet*, Nov 10, 1973, vol.2, pp.1053–5.

[32] R.K. Wallace, *The Physiological Effects of Transcendental Meditation*, Ph.D. Thesis, Dept of Physiology, University of California, Los Angeles, 1970.

[33] J.P. Banquet, 'Spectral Analysis of the EEG in Meditation', *Electrenceph. and Clin. Neurophys.*, 35: pp.143–151, 1973.

[34] J. Allison, 'Respiratory Changes During the Practice of the Technique of Transcendental Meditation', *Lancet*, no.7651, London, April 18, 1970, pp.833–834.

[35] Dr. P. Corey, 'Airway Conductance and Oxygen Consumption in Human Subjects via a Wakeful Hypometabolic Technique', National Jewish Hospital and Research Hospital, Denver, Colorado, April 1973, from the book: *TM-Discovering Inner Energy and Overcoming Stress*, H.H. Bloomfield MD, M.P. Cain, D.T. Jaffe, R.B. Kory, Unwin, 1975, pp.70–71.

[36] T. Routt, 'Transcendental Meditation and Relaxed States: A Pilot Study Comparing Physiological Parameters', ibid, p.82.

[37] R. K. Wallace & H. Benson, 'Physiology of Meditation', *Scientific American*, vol 226, no.2, Feb, 1972, p.88.

[38] R.K. Wallace & H. Benson, op cit., p.87.

[39] Ibid, p.90.

[40] E. Gellhorn & W.F. Kiely, op cit., pp.235–6.

[41] K.K. Datey, et al., op cit., pp.325–333.

[42] R.K. Wallace, H. Benson, A.F. Wilson, 'A Wakeful Hypometabolic Physiologic State', *American Journal of Physiology*, vol. 2221, no. 3, September 1971, pp.795–799.

[43] H. Benson & R.K. Wallace, 'Decreased Blood Pressure in Subjects Who Practice Meditation', Circulation, vols XLV & XLVI, October 1972 (Supplement 11). *Abstracts of the 45th Scientific Sessions.*

[44] S.G. Bandeen, *1948 Year Book*, Academy of Applied Osteopathy.

[45] T.L. Northup, 'Manipulative Management of Hypertension', *1957 Year Book*, Academy of Applied Osteopathy, p.43.

[46] T. Norris, 'A Study of the Effects of Manipulation on Blood Pressure', *1964 Year Book*, Academy of Applied Osteopathy, p.184.

ABOUT THE COMPILER

Dr Swami Shankardevananda
MBBS (Sydney)

- Born in 1952 in Sydney, Australia, he graduated in medicine in 1977.
- He came to Bihar School of Yoga, Munger, India as Chief Co-ordinator of the IYFM Research Co-ordinating Centre in 1974.
- While still a medical student, he met his guru, Swami Satyananda Saraswati in 1974, and was then able to alchemically blend the science of yoga and medicine into a unified system.
- He is the author of: *Yogic Management of Asthma and Diabetes, The Effects of Yoga on Hypertension, The Practices of Yoga for the Digestive System,* and *Amaroli.* He is presently working on the following books: *High Anxiety, The Principles of Yoga Therapy,* and *Yoga, Tantras and the Brain.*

INTERNATIONAL YOGA FELLOWSHIP MOVEMENT

A charitable and philosophical movement founded by Paramahamsa Satyananda at Rajnandgaon in 1956 to disseminate the yogic tradition throughout the world.

Medium of conveying the teachings of Paramahamsa Satyananda through the affiliate centres around the world.

Paramahamsa Niranjanananda is the first Paramacharya of the International Yoga Fellowship Movement.

Provides guidance, systematised yoga training programme and sets teaching standards for all the affiliated yoga teachers, centres and ashrams.

A Yoga Charter to consolidate and unify the humanitarian efforts of all sannyasin disciples, yoga teachers, spiritual seekers and well-wishers was introduced during the World Yoga Convention in 1993.

Affiliation to this Yoga Charter enables the person to become a messenger of goodwill and peace to the world, through active involvement in various far-reaching yoga related projects.

General Secretaries:
Sw. Satyabratananda 1956-1971.
Sw. Dharmashakti 1971 to present.

BIHAR SCHOOL OF YOGA (BSY)

A charitable and educational institution founded by Paramahamsa Satyananda at Munger in 1963 to impart yogic training to all nationalities.

Paramahamsa Niranjanananda is the Chief Patron of BSY.

Focal point for a mass return to the ancient science of yoga.

The original school, Sivanandashram, is the centre for the Munger locality.

Ganga Darshan, the new school, established in 1981, is situated on a historical hill with a panoramic view of the Ganges.

Yoga Health Management, Teacher Training, Sadhana, Kriya Yoga and other specialised courses are held throughout the year. Renowned for its sannyasa training and the initiation of female and foreign sannyasins.

Provides trained sannyasins and teachers for conducting yoga conventions, seminars and lectures tours around the world.

Has a well-staffed research library and scientific research centre.

Presidents:
Paramahamsa Satyananda 1963-1983.
Paramahamsa Niranjanananda 1983-1994.
Sw. Gyanprakash 1994 to present.

SIVANANDA MATH

A social and charitable institution founded by Paramahamsa Satyananda at Munger in 1984 in memory of Swami Sivananda Saraswati of Rishikesh.

Head Office now situated at Rikhia in Deoghar district, Bihar.

Paramahamsa Niranjanananda is the Chief Patron.

Aims to facilitate growth of the weaker and underprivileged sections of the society, especially the rural communities.

Activities include: distribution of free scholarships, clothing, farm animals and food; the digging of tube-wells and construction of houses for the needy; assistance to farmers in ploughing and watering their fields.

A small dispensary has been established for the provision of medicine, and veterinary services are also provided.

Tribhuvan Office, a three storey complex to deal with Sivananda Math's activities, will also house the satellite dish system for providing global information to the villagers.

All services are provided free and universally to everyone regardless of caste and creed.

Presidents:
Sw. Amritananda 1984-1987.
Sw. Haripremananda 1987-1989.
Sw. Siddheshwarananda 1989-1991.
Sw. Omkarananda 1991 to present.

YOGA RESEARCH FOUNDATION

A scientific, research-oriented institution founded by Paramahamsa Satyananda at Munger in 1984.

Paramahamsa Niranjanananda is the Chief Patron of the institute.

Aims to provide an accurate assessment of yoga practices within a scientific framework, and to establish yoga as an essential science for the development of mankind.

Conducted a symposium of over 100 medical professionals from India and abroad with a view to consolidating interest and work in yoga research and health investigation at Munger in 1988 and 1989.

At present conducting international research on the effects of yoga on respiratory disorders involving 10,000 subjects worldwide.

Future plans include literary, scriptural, medical and scientific investigations into other little-known aspects of yoga for physical health, mental wellbeing and spiritual upliftment.

Presidents:
Sw. Vajrapani, 1984 to 1989.
Sw. Gurukripa, 1989 to 1993.
Sw. Suryamani, 1993 to present.

SRI PANCHDASHNAM PARAMAHAMSA ALAKH BARA

Sri Panchdashnam Paramahamsa Alakh Bara was established in 1990 by Paramahamsa Satyananda at Rikhia, Deoghar, Bihar. It is a charitable, educational and non-profit making institution.

Upholds and propagates the highest tradition of sannyasa, namely vairagya (dispassion), tyaga (renunciation) and tapasya (austerity). Propounds the tapovan style of living adopted by the rishis and munis of the vedic era and is intended only for sannyasins, renunciates, ascetics, tapasvis and paramahamsas.

Alakh Bara does not conduct any activities such as yoga teaching or preaching of any religion or religious concepts.

The guidelines set down for the Alakh Bara are based on the classical vedic tradition of sadhana, tapasya and swadhyaya or atma chintan.

Paramahamsa Satyananda, who now resides permanently at the Alakh Bara, performs the Panchagni Vidya and other vedic sadhanas, thus paving the way for future paramahamsas to uphold their tradition.

Presidents:
Sw. Dharmashakti, 1990 to present.

BIHAR YOGA BHARATI (BYB)

The Bihar Yoga Bharati Institute was founded by Paramahamsa Niranjanananda in 1994 as an educational and charitable institution for advanced studies in yogic sciences.

It is the culmination of the vision of Swami Sivananda Saraswati and Paramahamsa Satyananda.

BYB is the first institute in the world of its kind to impart comprehensive yogic education with provisions to grant higher degrees in yogic studies such as MA, MSc, MPhil, DLit, and PhD to the students.

It offers a complete scientific, yogic education and training according to the need of the present times, through the Faculties of Yoga Philosophy, Yoga Psychology and Applied Yogic Science.

Residential courses of three months to two years are conducted in a Gurukula environment, so that along with yoga education, the spirit of seva (selfless service), samarpan (dedication) and karuna (compassion) for humankind is also imbibed by the students.

Vice-Chancellor:
Sw. Shankarananda, 1994 to present.